Thorsons Natural Health

Stomach Ulcers

Other titles in this series:

Arthritis
Asthma
Diverticulitis
Hayfever
Hiatus Hernia
High Blood Pressure
Prostate Problems
Skin Problems
Tinnitus

Thorsons Natural Health

Stomach Ulcers

LEONARD MERVYN

Thorsons
An Imprint of HarperCollins*Publishers*

Thorsons
An Imprint of HarperCollins*Publishers*
77–85 Fulham Palace Road,
Hammersmith, London W6 8JB

Originally published in *The Science of Life* series
Published as *Stomach Ulcers and Acidity* 1990
This revised edition 1997

9   7   5   3   1   10   8   6   4   2

© HarperCollins*Publishers* 1990, 1997

Leonard Mervyn asserts the moral right
to be identified as the author of this work

A catalogue record for this book
is available from the British Library

ISBN 0 7225 3557 0

Printed and bound in Great Britain by
Caledonian International Book Manufacturing Ltd, Glasgow

Dedicated to Sarah and Charlotte Waller

Contents

	Note to Reader	8
	Foreword	9
Chapter 1	The Digestive System	15
Chapter 2	Indigestion and Related Conditions	32
Chapter 3	Peptic Ulcers, Their Symptoms and Causes	52
Chapter 4	The Role of Hydrochloric Acid	76
Chapter 5	The Role of Infection in Peptic Ulcers	89
Chapter 6	Medical Treatments of Peptic Ulcers	98
Chapter 7	Natural Treatments of Peptic Ulcers	117
Chapter 8	Dietary Approaches to Peptic Ulcers	133
	Index	156

Note to Reader

Foreword

Stomach and duodenal ulcers occur as a culmination of rejecting Nature's warnings over a period of years. Ulcers in either the stomach or duodenum don't just happen, they are often the result of years of the wrong eating habits, worry or stress, or failure to cope with our modern lifestyle and ignorance concerning how our body functions and how we can best look after it.

Man was never intended to live in our huge 'civilized' cities in an environment which is foreign to his 'natural' habitat. For centuries, in our Western civilization, man lived in a rural or semi-rural atmosphere. Even the big cities of 100 years ago were small in comparison to the sprawling metropolises we know today. During the past fifty or sixty years life has become much more complex, complicated and hazardous as we continue to make what we choose to call 'rapid progress'. No longer do we obtain fresh milk direct from the dairy, but in bottles or cartons which may be a few days old or, if it has been subjected to ultra high temperature processing, it may be several months old. We eat more processed, ready prepared and takeaway foods. In Australia one leading dietitian has said that 'one third of all meals are prepared or eaten away from the home and the public don't know what they are getting'. On top of this, government statistics show that 25 per cent of all kilojoules (calories) available to the Australian public come from alcohol or sugar.

Studies in other developed countries show a similar trend. It is little wonder then that we see an ever-increasing incidence of stomach and digestive disorders. Our food is not what it used to be, and consequently we have paid the price of deteriorating health.

Not all progress is bad, however, and if we can adjust our way of living and our way of thinking to accommodate change we can do much to reap the benefits offered by our modern civilization without losing our health or the quality of life we have been accustomed to enjoy.

Stomach ulcers are usually carefully nurtured and grown with loving care by the sufferer who is usually totally ignorant of what he is doing. Before an ulcer develops there are usually warning signs, digestive upsets and minor discomfort for months and very often for years before the ulcer becomes apparent. It is by paying attention to Mother Nature's warning signs and by successfully overcoming minor digestive problems that more serious disorders including gastric and duodenal ulcers can be avoided.

The digestive tract can be broadly divided into four sections. There are the mouth and oesophagus (gullet), the stomach, the duodenum and small intestine and the colon or large bowel. The chemistry of these four sections varies alternately from alkaline to acid. The mouth and oesophagus are alkaline, the stomach is acid, the duodenum and small intestine are alkaline and the colon or large bowel is acid. It is imperative that each section maintains its normal alkalinity or acidity for normal digestion and that each stage of digestion be satisfactorily completed before the food passes to the next section for further processing.

Digestion begins in the mouth and if food is not chewed thoroughly and completely mixed with saliva before passing to the stomach, digestion in the stomach is impaired. Anyone who suffers with any digestive problem should chew their food for at least twice as long as they are accustomed to do. Remember that you cannot overchew your food. Eat at a leisurely pace and chew it well.

Food transit time through the digestive system is also important. The food only remains in the mouth for a few minutes. In the stomach it takes from 2½ to 5 hours before the food is ready to pass to the duodenum. It takes a further 3½ to 4½ hours for the food to pass through the duodenum and small intestine before it reaches the large bowel. It should then pass through the large bowel in another 12 to 15 hours, making a total transit time of about 20 hours. In our Western diet with its predominance of refined carbohydrates, alcohol, sugar and fat, transit time can be as long as 72 hours! This means that many toxins from waste products can be reabsorbed into the system giving rise to all manner of illnesses. It is also important to realize that over 90 per cent of nourishment from our food is absorbed from the first half of the small intestine, some 3 to 5 hours after we have eaten it. Little absorption occurs after the food has proceeded past this point.

Food transit time is influenced largely by the type of foods we eat and also by exercise. Physical exercise is essential to normal digestion and it is usually sedentary workers who suffer with digestive problems, although no one is immune from them, particularly if they eat their food quickly, wash it down with tea or coffee and visit the pub regularly after work. To maintain normal food transit time adequate fibre must be included in the diet, so too must a plentiful supply of fluids, preferably water. It is unwise to drink with meals. Most people who drink with meals do so because they fail to chew their food thoroughly and so have to wash it down instead of mixing it with saliva and enabling it to slip down the gullet easily. Drink twenty minutes after a meal, not while eating.

Our Western diet also contains an excess of fat, sugar and salt. These should be reduced but not excluded from the diet. Stimulants such as tea, coffee and alcohol should be avoided.

What happens once an ulcer has developed? How do we overcome it and prevent it from recurring? That is just what this book is all about. There are many simple, easy-to-follow measures which can be employed to assist ulcer sufferers. Correct diet, simple herbal remedies, overcoming stress and learning to live in our present-day environment are all important to the ulcer sufferer. The value of foods such as yogurt, herbs like slippery elm bark and liquorice, vitamins and minerals are all explained simply and clearly. If you do not have an ulcer this book will show you how to avoid it; if you are unfortunate enough to suffer with one then this book contains much valuable information to help you overcome it.

For completeness this book also brings to the reader's attention certain medical advances in the treatment of peptic ulcers and other gastric complaints. It is important that those suffering from ulcer complaints should be aware of these medical therapies, since most people will be offered them. Such new approaches do not detract from natural self-treatments to prevent and heal peptic ulcers, but in fact should complement them.

1

The Digestive System

Before we consider and discuss the various aspects of gastric and duodenal ulcers it is important to understand the whole process of food digestion. Not only is food subjected to a superbly controlled sequence of processing from the time it enters the mouth to its eventual excretion; at each stage digestive juices of the right type and make-up play their part in reducing the food to a form in which it can be absorbed and utilized by the body. We need a digestive system because food constituents as presented in the diet are complex substances that have to be reduced to simpler ones before the body can assimilate them. Basically, during the process, starches and sugar are digested or hydrolysed to the simplest sugar glucose. Proteins are reduced to their individual amino acids, some twenty or so in all. Fats and oils are emulsified then broken down to their constituent fatty acids and glycerol, which are partially re-combined after absorption to produce the type of fats that the body needs. Some of the glucose remains to be used as fuel for the workings of the body but most of it is built up into animal starch called glycogen which forms part of the fuel reserves, ready to be split once more into glucose when required.

The amino acids derived from the food are absorbed as such then combined by body processes to produce the proteins specifically for the human body. Some amino acids are set aside for other uses, for example, as brain and nerve transmitters; others can be utilized as fuel and inter-converted to make other amino acids. Fats represent a very important energy reserve since they are readily broken down and fed into the energy-producing cycle, like glucose, but they do have other specific functions. These are usually well catered for so that the problem is usually too much rather than too little fat laid down as energy storage depots.

It is relatively easy to break down the basic food constituents in the laboratory or in a factory. Boiling starches and proteins with acid will produce glucose and amino acids respectively. Boiling fats and oils with alkali will yield the free fatty acids (as sodium salts) and glycerol as in making soap. The digestive process is much less drastic although the end results are the same.

The body utilizes enzymes that are specific protein (organic) accelerators or catalysts that under certain conditions will break down the food constituents just like acids and alkalis do but in a more gentle manner. These enzymes require other constituents and narrow limits of acidity and alkalinity to digest food efficiently and the digestive processes are geared to supply these. Of course, digestive enzymes despite being proteins in structure, are not affected by the conditions under which they act in the digestive tract but are usually deactivated as they move through with the food at the next stage.

We shall now look at the process of digestion as it occurs at the various levels of the gastro-intestinal tract. The first stage happens in the mouth but even before food is introduced into it, various stimuli have caused the digestive juices to be produced. Even whilst the meal is being prepared, the smell of the cooking food, the thought of the taste to come and the anticipation of satisfying the appetite causes the saliva to flow. At the same time gastric juices, very potent in acids and enzymes, are secreted. Lower down in the twenty-two feet of small intestine other juices are being produced in readiness for the anticipated food. Apart from salivation the most obvious sign of the approaching meal is the gurgling of the stomach juices although this can be a symptom of hunger even without food in the offing!

The Mouth

The saliva produced by specific salivary glands in the mouth is there to lubricate the food and assist in the actions of chewing, cleaning the mouth and swallowing. In addition it contains an enzyme, ptyalin, that converts starches into maltose, a sugar that is almost at the ultimate stage of digestion. There is some doubt regarding the significance of this early digestive process since starch is readily digested further down the system. The efficiency of ptyalin depends upon how long the food is chewed; in animals that bolt their food, salivary ptyalin is absent.

The functions of the mouth and tongue are thus essentially to prepare the food for the main digestive processes further down the tract. They assist in the mastication of food and its formation into a bolus; they assist in swallowing. In addition the tongue is the sensory organ for the appreciation of taste, texture and temperature of food. Taste and texture are the stimuli to keep the digestive fluids flowing after their initial response to the smell of food.

These senses too are the first line of defence against eating food that is 'off'. The nose is the first to spot it and the usual reflex action is to spit out the obnoxious food. If some has already been swallowed both taste and smell will exert their protective actions by telling the stomach to refuse to pass the food on. The reverse process comes into play so the bad food is squirted back into the mouth from where it is readily vomited. The whole process is usually preceded by nausea so there is plenty of warning that the food is about to be rejected. Sometimes the food may have been passed on through the stomach to the intestine. This is usually the point of no return since there is a valve preventing intestinal contents from going back into the stomach. In such an instance the intestinal muscles will react by passing the poisonous contents quickly through the rest of the digestive tract. The end result is diarrhoea that disposes of the noxious material, eliminating it from the body. Hence although unpleasant, nausea, vomiting and diarrhoea are essentially protective and beneficial mechanisms.

The Oesophagus or Gullet

Although the oesophagus does not contribute to the digestive process, it links the mouth and the stomach. The walls of this connecting tube push the food into the stomach by a process of peristalsis which is simply alternating contraction and relaxation of the muscle. Gravity also contributes but peristalsis is the main process since thanks to this it is perfectly feasible to swallow when standing on one's head. There is some sort of valve, albeit not a very efficient one, between the oesophagus and the stomach so there is a little

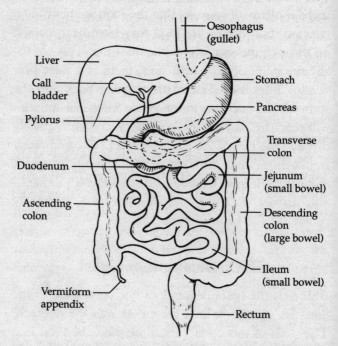

Oesophagus (gullet)

Liver

Stomach

Gall bladder

Pancreas

Pylorus

Transverse colon

Duodenum

Jejunum (small bowel)

Ascending colon

Descending colon (large bowel)

Ileum (small bowel)

Vermiform appendix

Rectum

Figure 1. The digestive system

Note the length of the duodenum, the long, narrow neck which connects the stomach to the small intestine. About 75 per cent of ulcers occur in the duodenum.

slowing down and control of the passage of food into the stomach. Usually however, the food passes fairly quickly into the stomach after swallowing. We shall see later how reverse movement of stomach contents into the oesophagus gives rise to a distressing condition called oesophagitis.

The Stomach

The stomach and the rest of the alimentary tract are shown in their relationships in Figure 1.

As the food is chewed the fluids produced by the salivary glands and the stomach continue to flow. The food is pulped with the teeth, tongue and the insides of the cheeks and mixed thoroughly with saliva. Eventually it is neatly packaged together at the back of the tongue where there are specific nerves that are stimulated to induce the act of swallowing. Once anything touches these nerves swallowing becomes an involuntary reflex action and nothing can stop the food or drink from entering the oesophagus.

Adjacent to the oesophagus is another entrance that leads down to the lungs or up into the nose. As food is swallowed a small soft body called the uvula rises to block off the nasal passages; at the same time the larynx (leading to the lung) is sheltered under the epiglottis so preventing food from entering the lungs. Food is thus directed down the oesophagus and as we have seen, it inevitably enters the stomach.

The stomach is of variable shape according to its contents and has the capacity to expand. It lies in the upper abdominal cavity, more to the right than the left. It is here that the digestive process really starts. Its action is like that of a washing machine where the pulped food gets turned over and over so that the various digestive juices can reach all parts of it. The walls of the stomach are rich in glands which secrete many substances. They include:

a) Mucin, a protein that acts to protect the walls of the stomach from acid.

b) Gastric juice which contains pepsinogen, which is inactive itself but is converted to the enzyme pepsin by another secretion, hydrochloric acid. Pepsin starts the breakdown of proteins. Another component, rennin, curdles liquid milk protein called caseinogen into the solid protein casein. This is then acted upon by pepsin.

c) Hydrochloric acid which creates an acid environment essential for the digestive enzymes to work. At the same time this acid can disinfect the food destroying harmful bacteria. It also destroys ptyalin the salivary enzyme. Hydrochloric acid also controls the pylorus which is the valve that functions between the stomach and the next length of small intestine known as the duodenum.

d) Hormones called gastrins are also secreted and they

have the function of keeping up the flow of gastric juice until the meal is digested. Gastrins also stimulate the release of intrinsic factor from the stomach walls and as we shall see later, this factor is absolutely essential for the absorption of vitamin B_{12}.

e) Lipases which help digest fats are also secreted in the stomach but their significance is doubtful since fat digestion is mainly the province of the intestine.

The stomach has a unique function not only as a processing chamber but also as a food store, for it has the capacity to expand to hold large quantities of food at a time. Drink that enters the stomach with food is passed on very quickly but some is mixed with the food, softening it further. Then it is squirted, a little at a time, into the next part of the gastro-intestinal tract, the duodenum. At this stage the stomach contents are known as chyme.

The Duodenum

The duodenum is about twelve inches long and is like a horseshoe in shape. It comprises the first part of the small intestine. It leaves the pylorus valve at the stomach and encircles the head of the pancreas to which it is firmly attached. It lies mainly to the right of the midriff and continuous to the next bit of the intestine called the jejunum.

The duodenum receives juices from two sources, the pancreas and the liver, via the pancreatic duct and bile duct respectively. Both juices are strongly alkaline so that in addition to their other functions they serve to neutralize the highly acidic chyme being squirted in from the stomach. The alkaline conditions that result in the duodenum act as the ideal medium in which the enzymes secreted in the duodenum can continue with the digestive process.

Pancreatic fluid is not only efficient in liquefying the partly digested proteins and the starches present in the food from the stomach but it has also the capacity to attack the fats in it. Bile assists in this because it contains bile salts, such as sodium glycocholate and sodium taurocholate, that emulsify fats and oils, rather like washing-up detergents that remove fatty residues from dirty plates.

The enzymes present in pancreatic secretion are:

a) Trypsinogen, inactive until converted to the active enzyme trypsin. This digests proteins and partly-hydrolysed proteins almost to amino acids.
b) Chymotrypsinogen, inactive until converted to the active enzyme chymotrypsin by the other enzyme trypsin.
c) Amylase, a starch-splitting enzyme that converts both starch and glycogen (animal starch) almost to glucose.

d) Lipase, a fat-splitting enzyme that causes hydrolysis of fat to fatty acids and glycerol. This enzyme is activated by bile salts which are produced in the liver and secreted in the bile.

e) Carboxypeptidase, secreted as inactive procarboxypeptidase but produced by the action of the other enzyme pepsin. The end result of carboxypeptidase digestion is some amino acids and combined amino acids called peptides.

The Small Intestine

The duodenum takes up only the first twelve inches of the small intestine. The rest is made up of the jejunum which is eight feet long and the ileum which comprises the last twelve feet.

Digestion is completed by enzymes secreted in the intestinal juices which are produced by the glands of Brunner and of Lieberkuhn. These enzymes are:

a) Aminopeptidase and dipeptidase which between them complete the digestion of proteins to simple amino acids.

b) Disaccharidases which complete the digestion of the products of digestion by amylases (pancreatic enzymes) to glucose.

c) Lipases that are specific for digesting complex fats like lecithin.

The small intestine, along its whole length, is also the main site for absorption of all the products of digestion which are now in a suitable state to be absorbed.

Hence the small intestine performs both digestive and absorption functions. It is often abused yet continues in its efficient manner. When we consider the hot spices; the unnatural cooked food; the overcooked or even burnt food items; the pips, stones, bits of paper, coins, even fragments of broken glass that we present the gastro-intestinal tract with, it is a miracle that the small intestine continues to digest and absorb. It can be polluted with medicines, alcoholic drinks, drugs, and infective microorganisms yet it still carries on.

In spite of these abuses the stomach and the small intestine and indeed the rest of the intestinal tract continue to work virtually twenty-four hours a day, churning up food, kneading it, mixing it with self-made juices, squirting it for hours on end until almost every constituent of the food has been reduced to its basics. These basics are glucose, amino acids, fatty acids, vitamins and minerals. The only constituent not reduced further is dietary fibre but even this has an important function, as we shall see later.

Absorption of these basic food constituents is an intricate process and the cells of the lining of the small intestine are particularly adapted for it. They comprise a highly specialized absorbing surface which is so finely and intricately folded that the total surface area is about that of two tennis courts! This is necessary because of the sheer volume of the food and digestive fluids passing down the small intestine. Every day we make almost three gallons of these fluids in order to digest our food and most of this volume has to be absorbed back into the body or we would die of dehydration. This is why we can continue to suffer from diarrhoea even after drinking nothing – in this case all the fluids are not absorbed. Persistent diarrhoea can be dangerous, particularly in babies and small children, because they are unable to replace the huge losses of water being excreted. This is why fluids are often introduced directly into the vein, to bypass the diseased gastro-intestinal system.

The stomach does not absorb anything apart from alcohol. This explains why the euphoric effect of alcoholic beverages is so rapid – absorption starts as soon as the stomach is reached. The ill-effects of alcohol appear much later because the body takes time to start disposing of the substance and it is the first metabolites like acetaldehyde that are toxic.

The Large Intestine

The large intestine, which is about six feet long, starts with the caecum which joins the end of the ileum at the ileocaecal valve. After this comes the ascending colon which bends at a right angle to continue as the transverse colon then turns through another right angle downwards to form the descending colon. The end of the colon (also called the large bowel) is the pelvic colon which joins to the rectum. This is the end of the line as far as food residues are concerned because the rectum ends in the anus, the excretory exit for the faeces.

The ileocaecal valve allows the food residues from the small intestine to go through into the caecum a little at a time. By this time the residues have less and less digestible material left with proportionately more of the indigestible plant fibre – cellulose and lignin – derived from fruit, vegetables and bran. In addition there is a very large quantity of bacteria present. These bacteria are the so-called 'friendly' ones that are beneficial to us, helping in the rotting-down process of the vegetable constituents in the food we eat. During this process they produce some B vitamins and the fat-soluble vitamin K. A proportion of these are absorbed so that we can make use of them and they contribute to our daily allowance of certain vitamins.

Strong antibiotics unfortunately kill these good bacteria, as well as the harmful ones, sometimes to such an extent that our intake of B vitamins and vitamin K is seriously reduced. For this reason these vitamins are sometimes prescribed with antibiotics.

If they are not, it is still useful for an individual to take a vitamin B complex product whilst on antibiotics and for a short period afterwards. Destruction of 'friendly' bacteria can also cause diarrhoea so freeze-dried preparations of them in powder form or even living yogurt can help by supplying fresh colonies.

The food has been digested and its nutritious components absorbed by the time it reaches the beginning of the large intestine. It is still however semi-fluid and the function of the large intestine is to extract most of the remaining water. This conservation of water in our body is important since if it were allowed simply to go through the rest of the system, dehydration would soon result. The mass of food residue plus bacteria is steadily pushed along the large intestine, losing more and more water along the way, and finally ending up as a solid mass. In this form it is stored near the end of the large intestine where accumulation takes place before the final excretion.

This mixture is now faeces and at a certain time, usually after breakfast, it is transferred *en masse* into the rectum. The rectum responds by telling the brain that it wants to rid itself of this material and the end-result is the desire to defecate or 'open the bowels'. Under normal conditions this is complete. The semi-solid faeces are extruded in the characteristic sausage form which in fact reflects the shape of the lining of the rectum. The act of defecation to completion immediately produces a strange feeling of well-being and satisfaction. At the same time it must be remembered that this material is not normally poisonous or harmful. It consists mainly of undigested fibre and harmless bacteria that can continue this 'rotting-down' process even after leaving the body. The brown colour of normal faeces is derived from bile pigments – the smell comes from the decomposition process caused by the 'friendly' bacteria.

Although most of the food constituents of our diet are digested then absorbed, the undigested fibre plays an important role throughout the digestive tract. Because they cannot be digested, fibres such as these found in bran, fruit and vegetables survive throughout the whole system and add bulk to the food contents. This bulk enables the whole of the gastro-intestinal system to carry out its peristaltic action in moving the food, even when mainly digested, along the tract. At the same time, these fibres absorb water and in so doing they swell, giving the walls of the gut a solid mass to work on. At the excretory end fibre is really important since its bulk and water-retaining capacity enable the faeces to maintain a semi-solid state. Constipation is due to over-absorption of water resulting in hard, compacted faeces; diarrhoea is the retention of too much water by the faecal mass. Hence dietary fibre can help by normalizing the water content of the excreta in both cases.

It seems that even soluble, indigestible food fibres like guar gum and other vegetable gums have an important part to play in the absorption and excretory systems. When dissolved in water, these gums act like a gel which also supplies bulk to the food mass. As gels they perform two very important functions. They slow down the absorption of sugars, so preventing a massive rise in blood sugar occuring after a meal. In addition they retain water and hence present bulk to the faecal constituents, aiding the insoluble fibres in their functions.

2

Indigestion and Related Conditions

There are many conditions associated with the stomach and adjacent parts of the digestive tract that can be a prelude to or consequence of gastric ulceration and excess acidity. These can be prevented or treated by sensible eating and care in the diet. Knowledge and correct diagnosis of these conditions and their early detection and treatment can often prevent the occurrence of the more serious peptic ulceration and its consequences.

Simple Indigestion

Eating too much denatured and processed food, eating too quickly, and eating badly prepared or ill-assorted combinations of food, can all bring on an attack of acute indigestion. This is also known as dyspepsia but no matter what it is called, it causes much discomfort. Sometimes this is relieved by vomiting which is Nature's way of curing it. More often though there is a very unpleasant feeling of nausea. Relief can be gained by drinking heavily salted water or, more drastically, by sticking two fingers down the throat. These heroic measures are not often needed however. Relief is often obtained simply enough by getting some cool, fresh air on the face or having a drink of cold water. Many people will experience a bloated, distended feeling often amounting to pain. One common cause is the result of air swallowed during the meal but it may also be due to nervousness. A meal that has lasted too long is often the reason. The best relief, embarrassing as it may be, is often a good belch. An attack of hiccups, though perhaps just as embarrassing, is usually the end-result.

For these symptoms there are many traditional remedies that are helpful – amongst the most pleasantly effective are the liqueurs taken at the end of a banquet. Originally this was why they were produced and drunk traditionally at the end of a meal and all are based on natural aromatic oils. Orange, peppermint, aniseed and dill are amongst the most popular and effective plant oils. Such oils are known as carminatives and in the hands of the herbalist are used extensively in the relief of flatulence. No one is quite sure how these oils in liqueurs settle the stomach but the alcohol content plays no part. Relief from flatulence is just as easily obtained from peppermints, orange slices, root ginger or essential oils from these plants. Just as important as taking this treatment is the half-hour rest after a heavy meal. In babies, gripe-water has the same carminative effect and it is worth remembering that this remedy can be just as effective in adults.

These treatments are all natural ones; to attempt to deal with the condition by taking strong medicine or alkaline powder is not the way to clear up the trouble. The price of purchasing a little momentary relief by these means is to render yourself more and more open to future attacks. Such treatment merely treats the effect. It makes no attempt to remove the cause which lies largely in our traditional feeding habits.

Both rich meals and alcoholic drinks have a de-hydrating effect, probably because, as we have seen, vast amounts of digestive juices are needed to cope with the food and the body will draw on its reserves of water to supply them. Alcohol, by virtue of its properties, will literally draw water out of the body tissues. The simplest remedy to ensure against suffering the day after over-indulging in food and drink is to drink not less than a pint of water before going to bed. This makes up the balance of the water previously lost and is the best natural treatment. As we shall see, however, it is simpler and better not to over-indulge but look more closely at what you eat and drink.

Occasional indigestion, particularly in the evening, can often be relieved by other natural means. Try getting extra sleep by going to bed early or getting up late. Take at least two hours exercise in the open by walking, golfing or gardening. Eat only light portions of food such as fish and fresh fruit. Carry on drinking large volumes of non-alcoholic drinks like natural, unsweetened fruit juices to keep down the calories but increase your vitamin C intake. In all circumstances avoid sleeping pills. Don't be misled by taking 'the hair of the dog' alcoholic drinks. This is a complete fallacy as it is now known that alcohol can only delay recovery. Give your digestive system a chance to recover – don't overload it with the very foods that caused the trouble in the first place.

There are always people who seem to develop indigestion easily and frequently, almost to the extent of daily discomfort. Often such attacks occur after consuming rich red wines, spices or citrus fruits. Although frequent attacks may give the individual the impression that there is something medically wrong, this is not often the case. It is a nuisance that can be prevented by sensible eating. It is often quite erroneously assumed by such individuals that they are allergic to these and other food items. Real food allergies are quite different and often result in copious vomiting, diarrhoea and skin reactions that give rise to blotchy, itchy rashes and patches. True allergy can make the unfortunate individual very ill indeed. Once allergies have been professionally identified, the only remedy is to avoid the food items causing them. Simple indigestion is only very rarely due to an allergy.

Nervous Indigestion

The simple indigestion discussed above can have a variety of causes including, as we have seen, allergies to food constituents. In addition to these physical causes however we must also add those due to psychological trauma. In this case nervous tension is often the culprit; a condition that can be brought on by stress, worry, external pressures or even an imminent examination, interview or some other event. Too often the immediate treatment is to take sedatives and tranquillizers to calm the nerves since these are the basis of the problem. This approach is most unwise since these drugs only create much worse problems of drug dependence, depression and drowsiness which in turn dulls the mind. Look instead to the cause of the nerviness. Self-examination may often be sufficient to rectify it. If you feel the need of a calming down agent, seek a herbal preparation or a high potency vitamin B complex formulation. These are mild, safe, non-habit forming and function through natural methods on the nervous mechanisms.

When we consider that we do not consciously tell

our digestive system to work it is obvious that to a large extent the nervous control of the whole digestive process is not under our own control. Nevertheless since nervous indigestion is a fact of life conscious thought can stimulate the flow of juices, perhaps when we don't need them, and contractions of the stomach and the rest of the digestive system. The nerves that tell our system these things reside in a large, multi-functional nerve called the vagus. This supplies many other organs of the body as well as the digestive tract so it is not surprising that mental factors can affect the workings of the stomach. In fact, one treatment for over-production of stomach acid and chronic indigestion is by cutting the vagal nerves that supply the stomach but this drastic therapy is now often replaced by less invasive treatments.

Chronic Indigestion

Many attacks of indigestion are temporary and giving the stomach a rest is often all that is needed for relief. Some people, however, do appear to suffer a constant discomfort after eating. This may be related to habitual wrong feeding and is aggravated rather than helped by the taking of one or more of the patent medicines on the market. Treatment therefore resides in a change in diet and it is gratifying to see how often this does the trick. This approach is dealt with later in the book but if, despite sensible eating, chronic indigestion persists it is sensible then to seek professional medical advice.

Heartburn

This is due to the acid stomach secretions regurgitating into the gullet, giving a burning sensation. This reflux of the stomach contents often happens when one is lying down after a heavy meal or even by bending down. Such heartburn is not unusual since it is simply related to the position of the body but if it happens in the upright position it means that the contractions of the stomach are actually pushing the acidic contents up into the gullet. They have managed to force their way through the ring of muscle between the gullet and stomach which, although not quite a sphincter or valve, usually manages to contract to hold the juices back. Although the stomach has an internal surface able to cope with acid, the oesophagus does not and it reacts by causing pain and burning sensation. The pain is known as heartburn and it is quite descriptive since it is frighteningly similar to the pain of some heart attacks. Again, if it happens only occasionally it may pass or it can be treated with a natural oil like peppermint but if it occurs consistently it should be treated by other means. It can be the cause of a disease called oesophagitis (see page 42).

People who are overweight have a greater tendency to suffer from heartburn. It can also happen in those with a malformation at the lower end of the gullet so that some of the stomach lies in the chest. This is called a hiatus hernia (see page 46).

Logical measures to reduce heartburn are weight reduction, avoidance of tightly constricted clothing around the abdomen, and stopping smoking. Sleeping position is also important. Elevation of the pillow on a 10-inch wedge is most beneficial in reducing acid exposure in the lower oesophagus. In view of their effects on the lower oesophageal sphincter, it is sensible to cut down on fat intake, avoid alcohol and coffee, and resist eating large meals late at night. These are general measures that have been proved successful in the majority of heartburn cases.

When heartburn becomes chronic many other foods, particularly spicy ones, may increase the pain and inflammation by directly irritating the inflamed lining of the lower oesophagus on their way to the stomach. Certain foods may also worsen symptoms by decreasing the force of the wave of muscle contractions that propel foods into the stomach. Some foods stimulate excessive production of stomach acid.

The following foods contribute to heartburn so it is best to try to avoid them if you suffer from the complaint: alcohol, chocolate, coffee, fatty foods, milk, orange juice, strong peppermint taken for long periods, strong spearmint, spicy foods, sugar, tea, tomato juice and other vegetable juices. In the short term both peppermint and spearmint can help to relieve heartburn, but too much taken for too long will exacerbate the problem.

Remember to drink plenty of water especially after meals if you suffer from heartburn. Water soothes the irritated oesophageal lining by flushing the mixture of food and stomach acid into the stomach. Small meals are less likely to cause heartburn, whereas large meals distend the stomach, causing strain on the oesophageal muscle. If you are overweight, this causes increased pressure in the abdomen. This in turn increases the tendency for the stomach contents to be pushed back up into the oesophagus and heartburn results. Try to lose those extra pounds.

Additional therapy which has been proved to be very effective is aimed at neutralizing or reducing gastric acid secretion with one of the new anti-secretory drugs (see page 101) all of which can be obtained, albeit at low potency, without prescription. Simple antacids may also help. However, be warned that such measures should only be undertaken on a temporary basis. As we shall see later, all have their disadvantages, and prolonged suppression of stomach acid can lead to more serious problems. Surgery is only of benefit in severe chronic heartburn that is due to a large hiatus hernia.

'Indigestion' due to Wind

Whenever food, liquid or simply saliva is swallowed air usually accompanies it. This is just ordinary air that happens to be in the mouth at the time of swallowing. There is vast individual variation in the amounts of air swallowed; some people swallow several gallons during the course of a day. Even new-born babies swallow air. At birth there is no air in their stomachs but it is introduced as soon as they are able to swallow. Suckling is notorious for introducing air into a baby's digestive system resulting often in pain and discomfort that can only be relieved by a burp.

Usually we do not notice swallowed air but you can guarantee that it is always there. Only when it reaches large volumes does it become uncomfortable producing a relieving belch. The problem is that we invariably swallow more air in preparing to belch, only to bring it up again.

Too often, it is possible to get into the habit of associating the occasional ordinary feeling of mild discomfort in the stomach with 'a little bit of wind'. Attempts to belch it up cause more air to be swallowed, more discomfort and the whole cycle to start again. The end result is a glorious belch that was totally unnecessary in the first place as air was introduced as a deliberate action. Ignore ordinary, occasional mild twinges in the abdomen and don't exacerbate the condition by introducing unnecessary air.

It is amazing how often it is believed that 'wind' forms in the stomach. It does not. All air within the gastro-intestinal system has been swallowed. One of the most common abdominal complaints in the world is that of 'wind' but it is not a disease and simply reflects the bad habit of swallowing air. Belching may be considered a compliment to the chef in some parts of the world but it never justifies a visit to a practitioner nor does it indicate a dietary or digestive disorder.

Oesophagitis

Oesophagitis (inflammation of the oesophagus or gullet), gastritis and peptic ulcers are responsible for the vast majority of indigestion pains and difficulty in swallowing. We shall therefore consider each in turn, but diagnosis of each particular complaint must be left to the practitioner.

The oesophagus is ostensibly a very simple structure but its mobility is similar to that of the gastro-intestinal system. At the top end it has a sphincter (or valve) that acts as a barrier to accidental swallowing because it is usually constricted, except when swallowing. The lower sphincter, connecting with the stomach, is less well defined but it is a barrier sufficient to prevent continual reflux (bubbling up) of gastric contents into the bottom end of the oesophagus. It is more of a kink than a developed valve but combined with a slightly higher pressure in the oesophagus it usually prevents regurgitation of stomach contents.

The lining of the oesophagus simply provides mucus to lubricate swallowing, rather like saliva does in the mouth. Although the lining of the lower end may secrete a tougher mucus to stand up to acid gastric contents it is not able to withstand them for long and the burning pain of oesophagitis is due to a direct action of this acid on the lining of the oesophagus.

The oesophagus is a relatively simple structure and there are only a limited number of mechanisms operating in its disorders. The most usual are physical obstruction, an inefficient valve, direct damage and bleeding. Obstruction may be caused by a foreign body; a growth; muscular uncoordination of the valve; a spasm or by a stricture or narrowing of the tube due to scar tissue from a previous injury. Sometimes the valve fails to relax or open and when this happens the main symptom is difficulty in swallowing.

An inefficient valve will allow the gastric contents to squirt up into the oesophagus, causing inflammation and pain. Damage to the oesophagus can be caused by swallowing any corrosive substance or, in some cases, medicinal drugs. The antibiotics tetracyclines, the anti-spasmodic drug emepronium bromide, and the mineral supplement ferrous sulphate are the main offenders but there are other drugs that can cause a similar inflammation if incompletely swallowed. Bleeding in the oesophagus can be due to a variety of causes but the most likely is scarring of the lining with sharp foods like crisps, crushed boiled sweets and the like. Oesophagitis is made worse by smoking and drinking alcohol. Coffee and popular drugs like aspirin can also exacerbate the condition.

Signs and Symptoms of Oesophagitis:

The two predominant symptoms of oesophageal disorders are difficulty in swallowing and pain. The cause of the pain is usually mucosal inflammation and is usually described by the sufferer as indigestion or heartburn. The pain is usually located behind the breastbone but it can radiate into the arms or neck. It is usually associated with meals or with certain foods; with posture, being intensified by bending forwards or lying back, and with the sensation of regurgitation, perhaps even into the mouth. These signs and symptoms are characterisitic of the condition 'reflux oesophagitis'.

If the pain is due to oesophageal spasm it is much less characteristic and more easily confused with the pain of a heart condition. It is, however, relatively rare. Loss of appetite and possibly nausea may also result from pain in the oesophagus, no matter what is the cause.

Bleeding from the oesophagus is very rare. However, any vomiting of blood is serious and requires medical attention. Unchanged blood, red in colour, suggests the origin of the bleeding is the oesophagus. On the other hand, partly digested blood that is colourfully described as 'coffee grounds' suggests it has arisen in the stomach or duodenum.

Difficulty in Swallowing (Dysphagia)

We have all experienced 'a lump in the throat' for emotional or other reasons and it makes swallowing difficult, uncomfortable or even painful. Anxiety and depression can cause the same sort of feeling and is often the reason for the 'relaxed throats' that are common in tense or nervous people. If the oesophagus is blocked or paralysed by disease however, it is possible to swallow quite easily but instead of carrying on down, the food stops moving and may be regurgitated into the mouth. Although sometimes secondary to pain, this type of difficulty in swallowing may be due to more sinister causes and professional help should be sought.

Hiatus Hernia

Hiatus hernia is a distinct anatomical defect where the sphincter between oesophagus and stomach is displaced from its normal site at the point level with the diaphragm where the oesophagus joins the stomach (see Figure 2). There are two types of hiatus hernia, the sliding type and the para-oesophageal type. These are also illustrated in the diagram.

In the sliding type of hernia, the top end of the stomach has slid up into the chest. The oesophagus empties into it perfectly well since the sphincter is well into the chest. Food goes down inside the gullet, past the diaphragm muscle and on into the intestine perfectly easily. The only discomfort in some people is that there is easy regurgitation of food back into the gullet from the stomach. The result is an acid heartburn pain just behind the breastbone after meals.

This sort of hernia is a minor problem and treatment of it is easy. If it is due to overweight, the painful regurgitation will stop once the individual loses weight. The reason is that once this happens the pressure inside the abdomen will no longer tend to force the food back up into the chest against gravity. Hence all meals should be small ones so that the food will go down easily and stay down. Another tip is to stay sitting upright for a few minutes after each meal so that the food stays down. When these relatively simple

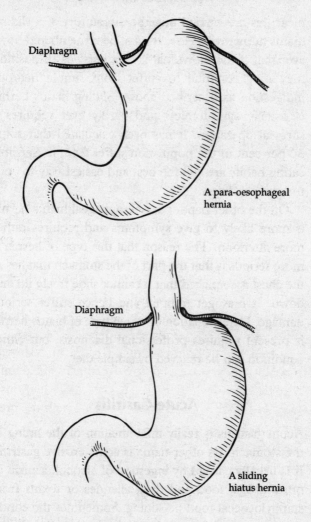

Figure 2. Types of hernia

measures are carried out, the discomfort of a sliding hiatus hernia will cease. It must be remembered however that if the individual is of a nervous disposition they may continue to suffer from simple nervous indigestion as described above. Sliding hiatus hernia is usually symptomless and hardly ever requires a surgical operation. It has been calculated that some 30 per cent of the population suffer from it. Sensible eating habits are still the best and easiest way to control the condition.

On the other hand, para-oesophageal hiatus hernia is more likely to give symptoms and requires rather more attention. The reason that this type of hernia is more serious is that the part of the stomach that lies in the chest is so placed that it cannot slide freely up and down. It may get trapped and hence suffer serious damage. Determination of which type of hiatus hernia is present requires professional diagnosis, but either condition can be relieved by simple diet.

Acute Gastritis

Acute gastritis is really inflammation of the lining of the stomach. Its other name is acute erosive gastritis. It is usually caused by ingestion of alcohol, aspirin or other drugs, food and drug allergies or toxins from staphylococcal food poisoning. Sometimes the condition accompanies such apparently unconnected diseases like those of the kidney and infections like influenza. Other causes include over-eating, the unwise combination of foods, or one or more of the dietetic indiscretions listed in this book. Usually gastritis is the stomach's definite indication that it can no longer tolerate the foolish and indiscriminate manner in which it has been fed and treated. It then proceeds to stage a strike against all further food until the whole digestive tract has been cleaned out – which is a somewhat painful and exhausting procedure.

Symptoms of acute gastritis are commonly lacking but loss of appetite, nausea, vomiting and gastric pain after eating may be present. Very occasionally the stomach lining may actually bleed. Treatment is usually aimed at withdrawing the offending agent, whether it is a medicinal drug or a food to which the sufferer is allergic. Changing the diet or ceasing to take alcoholic drinks will also relieve the condition. Fortunately the lining of the stomach regenerates itself very rapidly. Once the cause has been identified and removed, the self-healing process takes over and the stomach returns to normal after one or two days.

Corrosive Gastritis

This complaint is usually caused by swallowing strong acids, strong alkalis, concentrated iodine, potassium permanganate solutions or heavy metal salts like lead, mercury and cadmium. Gastric damage varies depending upon the nature and amount of the ingested poison. Often ulceration of the lips, tongue, mouth and throat will give a clue to the cause of the condition. Dysphagia or difficulty in swallowing suggests the oesophagus has also been damaged. The main symptom is severe abdominal pain sometimes accompanied by gastric bleeding.

The antidote and treatment depend upon the specific agent and amount taken and on the time interval before treatment. Acids are neutralized by alkalis and vice versa so here the antidote is fairly obvious. Other poisons may need expert advice, however, since induction of vomiting which may appear obvious may simply transfer the poison from the stomach to the gullet, throat and mouth where its corrosive action continues.

Chronic Gastritis

This is where the lining of the stomach is persistently inflamed but no one is quite sure what the cause is. Recent evidence suggests that the passing back or reflux of bile into the stomach is to blame. The bile acids have been particularly implicated in the condition since these are known to cause erosion of the stomach lining. Chronic gastritis is often a feature of gastric ulceration and in some cases may be the cause.

Hence the dietary suggestions to prevent and treat gastric ulcers that are discussed later (page 146) should also help in overcoming chronic gastritis. Apart from dietary treatment there is no other effective therapy for this distressing condition.

Dyspepsia

Dyspepsia is a condition in which the nerves of the stomach inhibit normal digestion and cause stomach acidity. Flatulence and gas pains are common. The typical dyspeptic is a neurasthenic. That is to say, his digestive troubles arise out of his restless, unrelaxed nature. He eats without discrimination at irregular intervals, leads a restless, ill-planned life, and subsists on a diet sadly deficient in all natural nerve foods and vitamins. He often smokes too much, drinks a lot of coffee, tea or spirits and fails to obtain sufficient sleep.

3

Peptic Ulcers, Their Symptoms and Causes

The number of people who suffer chronically from stomach or duodenal ulcers, acidity, dyspepsia or indigestion is appalling. No statistics are available, but unofficial estimates by medical practitioners are to the effect that one person in every three over the age of thirty is either a chronic or partial sufferer from some kind of indigestion, gastric upset, or ulceration of the digestive tract. The pain and misery of these people as the result of their meals cannot be computed in terms of unhappiness.

It has been estimated that some twelve per cent of the adult population of Australia suffer from a stomach ulcer or its forerunner, chronic indigestion, after every meal. In Britain, medical authorities have estimated the number of sufferers from these two stomach ailments to be in the vicinity of four million.

In the USA some authorities claim that as many as ten million people or more suffer from peptic or duodenal ulcers or acute, chronic indigestion. No club, no bar, no place where people meet is complete without its group of ulcer sufferers, and the doubtful humour which accompanies them. But ulcers are no joke. They are tenth among the list of chronic diseases as a cause of death and twelfth as a cause of absenteeism. American experts reckon that one out of every ten people is now bound to have a peptic ulcer sometime before they die.

Gastric ulcers occur mostly in early life. Duodenal ulcers usually pester middle age. Most ulcers are small – from a quarter of an inch to an inch in diameter. But they have an unpleasant habit of boring inwards through the walls of the stomach or duodenum rather than spreading along the surface. That's why ulcers kill. If they perforate those walls, you may die. Before we proceed, let us define the various types of ulcers to which human beings are vulnerable.

There are four times as many cases of stomach and duodenal ulcers among men than women, and for reasons which we will discuss later. The typical 'ulcer type' is generally lean, energetic, and anxious. Fat, placid men rarely get stomach ulcers. This is not to suggest that the lean, energetic type of person need get them – that to this type, stomach ulcers are inevitable. There is absolutely no need for any human being to become a victim of this painful – and highly dangerous – form of suffering that makes life a misery. Indeed, the suffering is incalculable, and the tragedy of it is that it is all so unnecessary. The consistent application of a few sensible principles can not only cure it, but can restore health to the highest level and keep it there.

What is a Peptic Ulcer?

Any ulcer is defined as an open, concave lesion of varying depth in the skin or mucous membrane. In the case of peptic ulcers, they are erosions through the mucous membrane that lines the gastro-intestinal tract, penetrating the muscular layer and even the blood capillary bed. Although we associate peptic ulcers with the action of stomach acid eroding the membranes, the digestive or 'peptic' enzymes also contribute. Hence the term peptic ulcer applies to those found in the stomach itself (gastric ulcer); the first few inches of the duodenum (duodenal ulcer); the lower end of the oesophagus (oesophageal ulcer), and that formed at the sphincter between stomach and duodenum, called a pyloric ulcer.

All types of peptic ulcer are the result of acid and peptic enzymes. The acid is hydrochloric, a strong acid that is needed for digestion, for sterilizing food that may be infected or water that is contaminated. It

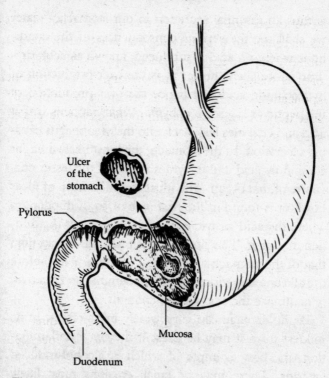

Figure 3. A stomach ulcer

An ulcer of the stomach, shown in the usual location, just at the pylorus, or exit of the stomach. The duodenum is shown below the stomach, and connects it with the small intestine.

The stomach of the average human adult secretes about three quarts of gastric juices daily. Gastric juices contain hydrochloric acid, pepsin and rennin. These digest food by chemical reaction.

is thus an essential secretion in our stomachs – later we shall see the serious consequences of the conditions where no acid is produced, known as achlorhydria. More likely, however, is the over-production of hydrochloric acid and hence the over-production of the peptic or digestive enzyme. What happens is that acid and enzymes leak back into the oesophagus causing ulceration. In the stomach, the most likely area for erosion by acid and enzymes is that of the lesser curvature of that organ. The most common form of ulcer however is found in the first inch or so of duodenum where the acid gastric contents first contact the duodenum lining. This lining is less resistant to acid than that of the stomach and erosion can take place before the alkaline secretions of the duodenum can effectively neutralize the acid gastric contents.

Peptic damage can vary widely in its effect. In its mildest form it may be present merely as inflammation, the best example of which is alcohol-induced gastritis. There may be small erosions most likely associated with certain drugs like aspirin and the anti-inflammatory medicines used in treating arthritis. The most severe form is a single large cavity that can reach half an inch in diameter, which is the classical peptic ulcer.

Since the gastro-intestinal tract has an inherent self-repair process, an ulcer is in a continuous state of flux with phases of damage and repair attending with each other. Examination by endoscopy (see page 61) hence reveals an inflamed active ulcer, full of exudate. In the quiescent repair stage that same ulcer appears as pale pink scar tissue.

The current view of peptic ulcer is that it is the result of an imbalance between normal erosive processes going on constantly and the ability of the tissue of the gastro-intestinal system to protect itself. Too much acid and digestive enzymes shifts the balance to the erosion side. In addition to these, however, must be included irritant drugs such as aspirin, anti-arthritic drugs, corticosteroids, iron salts, alcohol and bile. All of these can damage the lining of the stomach and duodenum.

What then are the protective factors? First and foremost is a thin layer of alkaline mucus secreted by the stomach lining. Production of this protective layer depends upon a healthy mucous membrane with the ability to have a fast turnover of cells to replace the inevitable losses. Replacement of these cells which produce the mucus, in turn depends upon various factors such as a good blood supply and protective hormones called prostaglandins. Both factors are the result of a good diet with an adequate supply of both vitamins and minerals so our food can play a big part in protecting us against peptic ulcers.

What are the Symptoms of an Ulcer?

The symptoms caused by ulcers are basically pain, the discomfort often making the sufferer belch as a result of trying to 'bring up the wind'. The pain is often quite characteristic in the way it comes and goes. Remember though that most instances of stomach pain have nothing to do with ulcers at all. These conditions were discussed in Chapter 2.

We have seen that the stomach can develop other disorders apart from ulcers even though the symptoms may be similar. The most common symptoms are loss of appetite, nausea, retching, vomiting and loss of weight. Even these can be due to emotional problems; disgust, for example, can easily cause nausea and vomiting; painful stomach cramps can arise from simple anxiety.

The usual symptoms of stomach ulcers are intense pain, vomiting and occasional haemorrhage. The pain is the most consistent symptom, and may come on from half an hour to two hours after eating. Those with duodenal ulcers experience exactly the same symptoms, only in their case pain is felt a little to the right of, and above the navel, instead of in the stomach itself. There is usually a longer time lag between the meal and the pain.

Here are some of the main easily recognized symptoms of ulcer:

- Chronic indigestion.
- Acid stomach.
- Acid belchings.
- Gas.
- Heartburn.
- Gassy distention.
- Burning sensation in the stomach.

In more severe cases these symptoms are present:

- Indigestion that appears about two hours after eating.
- Indigestion and stomach distress that suddenly stops when more food is eaten.
- Pain in the stomach.
- A sore spot in the stomach that is tender to pressure.
- Vomiting.
- Haemorrhage.
- Black-coloured stools. (They are black because of stomach haemorrhage.)
- Yellowing of the skin. (Caused by absorption of blood substance mixed in the food from bleeding ulcers.)
- Anaemia from loss of blood.

Of course, all of the symptoms may not be seen in every case of stomach ulcer but any one is a very suspicious indication that an ulcer is at work. Pain after meals is the most common and most certain symptom.

New York Specialist on Ulcer Symptoms

Dr Joseph F. Montague, a noted New York specialist, wrote the following useful outline of the symptoms of stomach ulcer and duodenal ulcer:

Stomach or duodenal ulcer starts a warning signal swinging in nine cases out of ten. That warning is pain, and the ulcer patient gets it invariably at some time of the day or night, if not at both of these periods, in the form of a sharp feeling of distress or a gnawing sense of discomfort. Whatever form the pain manifests itself in, it is well to heed it, for with ulcers generally an ounce of the good old prevention is worth the traditional pound of cure.

Very often when symptoms of so-called indigestion appear, the patient doses himself with this or that nostrum, or contents himself with taking a nightly purge. In the minds of many men there persists the belief that a physic will cure practically every ailment of the human body. So, the stomach ulcer patient, conscious of a burning sense of distress in his stomach, beneath his breast bone or between his shoulder blades, takes this or that laxative in the naive belief that he can wash his trouble out of him. Such purgatives are a positive menace where an ulcer is present, for they irritate tissue and stimulate peristalsis to a point that causes bleeding.

Duodenal ulcer, on the other hand, often has little effect upon the patient's weight. His appetite remains fairly normal and his only awareness of trouble in his digestive tract is the distress that comes along after he has eaten, or when he is about to eat again.

How Ulcers are Located

To find out if you have an ulcer, a doctor will probably test the contents of your stomach before and after eating, and X-ray your stomach before and after you have eaten barium, which has a metallic content and therefore shows up on an X-ray photograph. If you have a chronic, deep ulcer the barium, an opaque substance, will fill up the hole the ulcer has left and reveal it. But it won't show up all ulcers, so your doctor may be left guessing whether that strange mark on your X-ray plate means that you have an ulcer or that you just have some kind of irritation.

With the increase of ulcer cases, medical science has devised a clever way of looking into the stomach. This is called endoscopy. Scientists have produced a flexible tube with a system of lenses and electric lights and tiny mirrors which can be swallowed quite easily. It allows the operator to see inside the stomach, and even to take coloured photographs. A normal stomach has thick, smooth, orange-red folds. An ulcer looks like a small volcanic crater set in a red plush curtain!

Incidentally, most ulcers – three out of four – occur in the duodenum. The duodenum is the narrow neck of the stomach which connects it with the small intestine. Also, ulcers are more frequent among men than women, due chiefly to the fact that during their middle years, their stomach acid reaches a higher level. They eat more rapidly than women, and are more likely to wash their meal down with tea, coffee, or beer, which are all acid-forming.

The Differences Between Duodenal and Gastric Ulcers

The causes of both types of ulcer are fundamentally different. Lack of the mucosal protection is the prime cause of gastric ulcers. When combined with irritation and inflammation of the stomach lining induced by various factors, a resulting ulcer is almost inevitable. The lack of a good blood supply to an area of the gastric mucous membrane also probably plays a part.

Duodenal ulcers are more likely to be a result of overexcretion of acid and peptic enzymes. The contact time between the duodenal lining and the erosive contents of the stomach as they pass into the duodenum also determines the susceptibility to duodenal ulcers. This can be prolonged for a variety of reasons and the chances of ulceration are increased. The effect of chronic stress is associated more with the development of duodenal than with gastric ulcers. Acute stress is more likely to cause gastric ulcers.

The pain of duodenal ulcers is often relieved by food; that of the gastric type is aggravated. Night pain is more a feature of duodenal ulcers. The development of cancer can be a feature of gastric ulcers but there is no association between it and duodenal ulcers.

Risk Factors for Peptic Ulcers

Stress remains one of the most important factors for the development of so-called 'acute stress ulcers'. The term embraces not merely psychological stress but also the metabolic stresses associated with severe illness, burns, surgery, and accidental injury, all of which can produce peptic ulceration as a secondary feature. Other factors include smoking, group O blood, drugs and a family history of gastric or duodenal ulcers. Although stress and medicinal drugs, because of their irritant action, may seem to be understandable factors, we are still uncertain as to why men are three times more prone than women to develop peptic ulcers. Nor do we understand why duodenal ulcers are three times as common as the gastric type. The fact that some 5 per cent of the gastric ulcers become cancerous whilst duodenal ulcers rarely do is another mystery.

What are the Causes of Peptic Ulcers?

There are many causes, and most victims have for many years been guilty of not one, but several of the following:

- Over-eating.
- Worry.
- The use of aluminium cooking utensils.
- Too much starchy food.
- Incompatible food combinations.
- Vitamin and mineral deficiencies.
- Mixed, messy and indiscriminate feeding.
- Hasty eating and improper mastication.
- Condiments.
- Sugar consumption.
- The laxative habit.
- Alkaline powders.
- Weakened resistance of the blood to noxious bacteria.

These causes are not necessarily listed in order of importance, and generally a combination of several of them is responsible for the ulcer. Let us examine them in some detail:

1. Over-eating:

Most people eat more food than they need for energy and the repair and maintenance of bone and tissue. All excess food puts an added strain on the digestive mechanism. Often it breaks down under the strain, and digestive troubles result.

2. Worry:

The brain and the stomach are connected by the vagus nerve. Tests have shown that when a person is worried the flow of the powerful gastric juices in the stomach is increased. Indeed, under such conditions it continues to flow, whether food is present in the stomach or not. If there is the slightest ulceration in the stomach, the constant flow of the gastric juices – which contain hydrochloric acid – irritates the ulceration and enlarges it. On this point, Dr Richard Harrison has written:

> The stomachs of people with severe nerve weakness are in a constant state of irritation and unrest.
> This is because the nerves that stimulate normal stomach activity do not stop working when the stomach is empty.
> Instead, a continuous flow of irritating stomach juices is produced. On the walls of an empty stomach this continual, unnatural flow of stomach juices has a damaging effect.

The stomach, after all, is a piece of meat. And stomach juices are designed to digest meat (and other protein foods).

Under ordinary conditions, Nature furnished good protection for the stomach tissues against its own juices. But when stomach tissues are continually saturated with a wholly abnormal amount of digestive fluid, some areas lose their protection ability ... An ulcer or ulcers is the result.

The destructive emotions of anger, rage, hate, jealousy and fear all have disastrous effects upon digestive processes. Meals eaten under mental or emotional tension lead to inadequate mastication, giving rise to faulty digestion. Worry and anxiety interfere with normal digestive activity.

3. The Use of Aluminium Cooking Utensils:

Aluminium is a soft metal, readily affected when used for cooking foods because it is soluble in both acids and alkalis. Most foods have either an alkaline or acid reaction.

Traces of oxide of aluminium, when combined with sodium chloride (common salt) from the cooking of vegetables in salt water, and ingested with food, adversely affect the health-giving potassium in the human body. There is also evidence that these tiny particles of aluminium enter the stomach and weaken the stomach lining with their astringent properties, thus encouraging the formation of ulcers.

4. Too Much Starchy (and Protein) Food:

Processed and refined starchy foods – bread, flaked, puffed and toasted cereals, porridge meals, cakes, pies, biscuits, rice, macaroni, etc. – constitute the bulk of the diet of the vast majority of the population. Both processed, starchy foods and proteins are acid-forming and an excess of these foods in the diet upsets the proper acid-alkaline balance and leads to acidity – the forerunner of all digestive troubles (and, incidentally, of rheumatism and arthritis).

Alkali-forming foods, which are more desirable, include vegetables, fruits and most nuts, apart from Brazils and peanuts. Remember, however, that foods are acid- or alkali-forming only after absorption and assimilation by the body. Whilst in the digestive system, fruits, for example, contribute citric, malic and other acids. Although these are weak compared with the strong hydrochloric acid that the body produces itself, they do contribute some acidity.

The important point about food and the diet in general is to ensure that each meal is balanced. Food constituents themselves, particularly the proteins, have a neutralizing or buffering action on stomach acids that can help prevent the effects of over-production. There is no such action by starches and sugars.

5. Incompatible Food Combinations:

Although a balanced meal, in respect of its various food constituents, is considered to be highly desirable by some authorities for the prevention of digestive problems this is not agreed for everyone. There is a school of medical thought which attributes much of the digestive troubles of men and women to the common practice of eating protein and starch foods, or acid and starch foods, at the same meal.

The starches referred to are – bread, packeted cereals, porridge meal, pastries, biscuits, jams, ice-cream, etc. These starch foods do not combine well in the stomach with protein foods (meat, fish, eggs and cheese) or with acid fruits (oranges, grapefruit, tomatoes, pineapples, peaches, plums, apples, apricots, etc.). This kind of 'incompatible feeding' often leads to gas, fermentation, flatulence, pain, and finally to chronic indigestion, dyspepsia, and/or ulceration.

The most sensible advice, however, is to be 'middle of the road' when it comes to eating meals, i.e. moderation in all things without excessive intake of any one particular food item, no matter how good you may think it is.

6. Vitamin and Mineral Deficiencies:

It is no exaggeration to say that 90 per cent of the entire population suffers from vitamin and mineral deficiency of some sort. If this were not so, there would not be over 3,000,000 admissions to public and private hospitals every year in Australia, for example, and people would be far healthier.

In the case of digestive and ulcer sufferers, there is abundant evidence that these unfortunate people have long been deficient in vitamins A, B complex, C and E, and in calcium.

Vitamin A is required for the health of the epithelial tissue (i.e. the inside of the mouth, the tonsils, trachea, lungs, intestines, lymphatic glands, and the walls of the stomach, pylorus and duodenum). This vitamin has been shown in medical trials to be effective in accelerating the healing of peptic ulcers (see page 124).

The B complex vitamins are essential to the health of the nervous organization and the secretion of enzymes necessary for good digestion.

Vitamin C is required for healing any ulcer. Vitamin C builds healthy connective tissue and strengthens the walls of blood vessels. It also helps to stimulate 'antibodies' and phagocytes which destroy bacteria in the blood-stream.

Vitamin E acts most beneficially upon the heart and muscles. It dilates the capillaries and permits an improved flow of blood to congested areas. It also dissolves blood clots. Lack of this vitamin in the ordinary diet appears to have some bearing upon the increase in the number of stomach ulcers.

Calcium is important to the health of the body. Without it, the nerves and muscles cannot relax, giving rise to tension. Without Vitamin D (which we mostly obtain from sunshine) and phosphorus, the body cannot utilize the calcium in our food supply.

7. Mixed and Indiscriminate Feeding:

Most of us have grown up in the evil dietetic tradition that all so-called food is good for us – that it's all 'grist for the mill'. We therefore proceed to eat anything and everything that comes our way, regardless of the appalling task we have set our digestive organs, our eliminatory organs, and the chemistry of the body itself. Soup, meat, vegetables, puddings, washed down by tea or coffee – down it all goes! We may feel satisfied after such a meal but we have set in motion the ingredients which finally create fermentation, flatulence, acidity, hyperacidity and stomach trouble. If that were not bad enough, our next meal may add to the offence by consisting of one or other of the doubtful concoctions found in the delicatessen shop. Here we see a picturesque assortment of embalmed, preserved and demineralized products, masquerading as 'food' in the form of pies, pastries, pickled pork, pickled onions, corned beef, pigs' trotters and an assortment of sausagemeats, consisting of meat scraps, flour, fat, colouring and artificial flavouring and seasoning. All these products are alleged to feed you, but in reality they will hasten the onset of the pains of stomach ulcers and ill health.

A generation less notorious for its educated ignorance would condemn all such foods as unfit for human consumption. Very hot drinks, highly spiced foods and ice-cold drinks and foods all irritate the stomach lining. Sufferers from stomach troubles should also abstain from alcohol which increases the acidity of the stomach.

8. Hasty Eating and Improper Mastication:

Every one must surely realize the digestive troubles they are inviting by eating meals under mental tension, leading to improper mastication and digestion. It is recognized by medical science that worry, anxiety and stress interfere with the normal activity of the stomach and that anger, rage and fear tend to over-excite and over-activate the flow of gastric juices.

9. Condiments:

A further potent cause of ulceration is the habit of taking condiments. We have come to depend upon the artificial stimuli of mustard, pickles, pepper, chutney, tomato sauce, salt, etc., to give us an appetite. But all these products are harmful irritants. They certainly stimulate appetite by exciting the flow of gastric juices but it is unnatural stimulation. The result is to leave the appetite more jaded than ever, so more stimulants are used, and so on. The result is that the lining of the stomach is subjected to such irritation that it becomes inflamed and finally ulcerated.

10. Sugar Consumption:

Sugar, whether white or brown is a refined, concentrated carbohydrate completely divorced from all the beneficial elements of the original sugar cane. It is sweetness without sustenance, devoid of the essential vitamins and minerals. Molasses, the residue of sugar cane, has nutritional virtues. But sugar is left with only the dangerous delusion – the highly refined crystals that please the eye, seduce the palate and increase acidity. But in spite of its pleasant appearance and taste, sugar is a slow, insidious poison, robbing the body of its calcium by neutralizing it, setting up fermentation and acidity, and slowly but remorselessly undermining the health of its host. If you value your health, don't use sugar. If you want a substitute, use honey, which contains both vitamins and minerals.

At one time, it was usual to over-emphasize the factors of stress and strain as the dominant cause of stomach ulcers. However, research done in the 1960s showed that there are fewer ulcers among top-ranking businessmen than among lower paid people doing routine jobs. The survey found that shift workers in particular are very prone to ulcers. It is also revealed that there are more stomach ulcers among townspeople than country dwellers, not because there is more stress in town living, but because townspeople eat more sugar. Moreover, stomach ulcers are now not uncommon among children, doubtless due to an unbalanced diet containing a high proportion of sugary foods, refined cereals, soft drinks, sweets, ice-cream, chewing gum, etc. More attention than ever before is now being directed to faulty nutrition as the real cause of stomach ulcers.

11. The Laxative Habit:

The taking of laxative pills and medicines is a notorious contribution to ulceration and inflammation of the digestive tract, especially the stomach. These laxatives are irritants; foreign bodies, which cause fermentation and unnatural stimulation of the nerves, muscles and mucous membrane of the stomach and alimentary tract. One authority explains their internal reaction as follows:

> When a purgative of any kind is introduced into the system, its presence is a constant irritation to the sensitive mucous lining of the bowel. The intestines react against the purgative, and in forcing it out of the system a bowel action necessarily takes place. But mark the fact that the action is brought about by the expulsion of the salts, or whatever it is, which the body regards as something foreign and repugnant to it.

It is now known that the regular use of laxatives can give rise to serious, even incurable, intestinal ailments in later years. Proper feeding will bring about regular bowel movements without pills or purgatives and the evils they lead to in the digestive system.

12. Alkaline Powders:

Sufferers from digestive troubles or stomach ulcers usually seek refuge in one of the antacid powders or bicarbonate of soda preparations on the market. They feel that because these alkali powders give some relief from the pain and flatulence which follow every meal, they must be counteracting the acidity and so assisting in the healing of the ulceration. This is not the case however. The antacid powder or bicarbonate of soda habit will in time make the condition worse. It does nothing to remove the cause of the trouble.

Dr William Howard Hay was once asked if antacid powder or bicarbonate of soda should ever be used to relieve indigestion or 'sour stomach' and he replied:

Not if used to correct stomach acidity, for it would aggravate the very thing for which relief was intended. Sour stomach comes from either an over-supply of hydrochloric acid or from the various fermentations of the carbohydrate foods (starches and sugars).

If from too much of the stomach acid mentioned, then correction by the soda merely means that enough or more of this acid will be secreted to continue the interrupted protein digestion, thus increasing the habit of formation of this, while if due to fermentation, this merely neutralizes the acids without in any way stopping the fermentation, which proceeds at the old rate.

The B complex vitamins, vitamin C, calcium and iron all need an acid medium in the stomach in which to carry out their various functions in promoting bodily health. Bicarbonate of soda, antacid powders and other alkalizers produce an artificially alkaline condition in the stomach, thereby neutralizing the action of the vitamins and minerals which are lost to the body.

13. Weakened Resistance of the Blood to Noxious Bacteria:

This is the logical outcome of nutritional deficiencies and defects in the mode of life, so usual with the digestive and ulcer sufferer.

4

The Role of Hydrochloric Acid

If you look up a chemistry text-book you will see hydrochloric acid described as a colourless fuming aqueous solution of hydrogen chloride gas with a very pungent odour. Yet this same acid in a dilute form is an important part of the human digestive system and its excess or lack can have profound effects upon the health of the individual. When too much is produced the condition is known as hyperacidity and this is one of the factors contributing to the formation of peptic ulcers. When too little is formed, the condition is called hypoacidity and the net result can be less effective digestion in the stomach. In some cases no acid at all is produced and the condition is referred to as achlorhydria. The absence of hydrochloric acid will increase the chances of developing gastric cancers.

Before we consider these various aspects of hydrochloric acid production, let us see how it is made within the stomach.

The Production of Hydrochloric Acid

In the lining of the stomach there are two types of secretory glands. One consists of a single layer of secreting cells known as chief cells which produce digestive enzymes. The other type of secretory gland consists of cells arranged in layers. They are known as parietal cells which secrete hydrochloric acid directly into the gastric glands and hence into the stomach. The mixed secretion is known as gastric juice. It is normally a clear, pale yellow fluid of high acidity, (between 0.2 and 0.5 per cent hydrochloric acid) but with 97 to 99 per cent water. Also present are the protective protein mucin, inorganic salts and digestive enzymes.

Hydrochloric acid is a combination of hydrogen ions (which determine acidity) and chloride ions. Hydrogen ions arise in the following manner. Carbon dioxide which is present in blood plasma as a normal respiratory component passes into the parietal cell. This cell has blood plasma on one side with the opening of the stomach on the other. Within the cell there is an enzyme, called carbonic anhydrase, which catalyses the reaction between carbon dioxide and water to form a weak acid known as carbonic acid. This is the same acid that is formed in carbonated drinks like lemonade. Because it is weak, carbonic acid readily dissociates into bicarbonate plus hydrogen ions. Bicarbonate cannot leave the parietal cell to enter the stomach but readily passes back the other way into the blood. The second component of hydrochloric acid, chloride, is always present in the blood (this is why blood tastes salty) and readily passes through the parietal cell and into the stomach itself. Here it combines with the hydrogen ions already produced by this specific cell and the net result is free hydrochloric acid.

Bicarbonate is alkaline and, as we have seen, this passes back into the blood. Hence after a heavy meal when hydrochloric acid is produced in great quantities, a lot of bicarbonate is also formed at the same time. This upsets the balance of acids and alkalis in the blood and it is then up to the kidney to restore the balance by getting rid of the extra bicarbonate into the urine. The end-result is the so-called alkaline tide which simply means that the urine is alkaline instead of slightly acid as normal. Alkaline urine promotes bacterial growth so too many 'alkaline tides' can eventually give rise to urinary infections.

Why Do We Need Hydrochloric Acid?

This acid, along with some weaker organic acids that are also secreted into the stomach, provides the right sort of acidity that is essential for the first digestive enzymes to work. The digestion of proteins starts under the influence of the enzyme pepsin which cannot function unless the pH (measure of acidity) is between 1 and 2. Hydrochloric acid is essential for the gastric juices to reach this low pH (anything below pH7 is acid and the stronger the acid the lower the pH).

There is another enzyme, also secreted by the stomach, that requires a very acid medium in which to work. This is rennin and its main function is to coagulate milk into a solid form that can be acted on first by pepsin then by other enzymes further along the gastro-intestinal tract. Lack of hydrochloric acid will therefore make milk more difficult to digest.

It must be pointed out, however, that those people who have had the whole stomach, or just that part that produces acid, removed are still able to digest proteins and milk. Their digestive processes may not be quite as effective as they would be with a normally functioning stomach but it does suggest that the roles of pepsin and rennin are not quite as critical as was once thought.

The presence of hydrochloric acid, however, becomes of prime importance in the liberation of vitamin B_{12} from food and its eventual absorption. In meat, which is the most important provider of B_{12}, the vitamin is attached to proteins and the prior digestion of these proteins is essential for the vitamin to be released. Once it is free, vitamin B_{12} is able to combine with a specific protein called intrinsic factor that is also produced in the parietal cells of the stomach.

This complex of vitamin and intrinsic factor can only be formed in the presence of hydrochloric acid and calcium. Once formed, the complex is then transported intact to the ileum where it is absorbed. If intrinsic factor is not present, vitamin B_{12} cannot be absorbed and the result is the once-fatal disease called pernicious anaemia. Lack of hydrochloric acid will therefore reduce the absorption of vitamin B_{12}. It is not without significance that a major symptom of pernicious anaemia is a complete absence of hydrochloric acid in the stomach.

Increased Secretion of Hydrochloric Acid

We can now look at the factors that can cause an increased secretion of hydrochloric acid and its consequences. Of all the digestive tract, the stomach is one organ which is relatively easy to get at and its response can be studied by observing it in people who by reason of accident or design have a hole in the stomach, known in medical circles as a gastric fistula. The strength and quantity of hydrochloric acid produced by the gastric cells can thus be measured under a variety of conditions.

Psychological moods were found to be amongst the most influential factors in producing excess hydrochloric acid. Anger, worry and anxiety all caused the stomach walls to become red, swollen and inflamed with a marked increase in movement and gross oversecretion of acid. Other studies indicated that similar symptoms became apparent when the person was disgusted, resentful, depressed, fearful or when there was a reason to feel insecure, hopeless or defeated. Significantly, the recall of past frustrations or disappointments alone was sufficient to stimulate excess acid production.

As we have seen, hydrochloric acid secretion is usually the response of the stomach to an anticipated meal. The rumblings and gurgles associated with hunger are the stomach's reactions to the expected influx of food. Once it is eaten, though, the first-secreted hydrochloric acid is neutralized but secretion continues in order to maintain an acid medium.

Certain constituents of food have been found to be more stimulating to acid production than others. High protein foods like meat and fish, and beverages like coffee and tea all have a profound stimulant effect on acid secretion. Bitter materials have been known for years to have a stimulant effect on the appetite; now we know that aperitifs like sherry and campari simply act by causing hydrochloric acid to be produced.

Despite popular belief, highly spiced foods like chilli, curry, pickles, vinegar, soused herrings, mustard and frankfurters have little or no effect upon hydrochloric acid secretion. The burning sensation suffered by some people on taking these foods is more likely due to a localized effect of the 'hot constituents' on the lining of the stomach.

In view of the corrosive action of the highly acidic gastric juice, and the exposure of the stomach mucosa to it, perhaps it is surprising that this lining does not break down more often. If it does, of course, the result is a gastric ulcer. Usually, however, the stomach is able to protect its lining by secreting large quantities of mucus. This mucus forms a tough barrier and confers a high level of protection. It is quite possible that people who suffer from gastric ulcers produce only a thin, weakened type of mucus or possibly none at all.

Even when the ulcer has formed, if a thick layer of mucus covers it, it cannot be attacked by stomach acid and often the gastric lining is then able to heal itself effectively. A traditional remedy for treating gastric ulcers is liquorice and this has been found to act by stimulating the production of a thick layer of mucus over the area of the ulcer. A widely-used drug called carbenoxolone that is successful in healing ulcers is derived from liquorice.

Other treatments for excessive hydrochloric acid production are simple neutralization with alkalis. Specific drugs and surgery are also used to control the acid production. Surgery involves cutting the nerve, called the vagus, which carries the impulses telling the parietal cells to make acid. Another approach is to use drugs that are known as histamine H_2 receptor antagonists. Since the naturally-produced histamine is a potent stimulator of hydrochloric acid production in the parietal cells, it is logical to use drugs that specifically block the action of histamine upon these cells. Hence acid production is curtailed and in its absence the irritant action is lost and the normal healing processes of the body are allowed to take over and get rid of the ulcer.

We shall see later how too little gastric hydrochloric acid can have serious consequences so it is possible that prolonged reduction in the secretion of acid by surgery or by drugs will increase the chances of these consequences. In a similar manner, constant neutralization of the stomach acid with oral alkalis can have serious effects: first by removing all of the acid so that the desired acidic medium in the stomach is lost; second because neutralization simply stimulates further production of acid so that more alkali must be taken and so on. A vicious circle is set up so that eventually the parietal cells simply give up.

Deficiency of Hydrochloric Acid

A deficiency or complete lack of stomach hydrochloric acid has more far-reaching consequences than an excess. Dietary minerals are solubilized by the acid and this makes them more amenable to absorption. Adelle Davis reported how an orthopaedic specialist found that his patients consistently had low levels of hydrochloric acid. Once the deficiency was overcome by supplementing with the acid, the rate of bone healing and ossification increased as more calcium became absorbed.

She also quoted references supporting the fact that an insufficiency of hydrochloric acid can result from a low intake of protein and deficiency of vitamins A, B_1, B_2, B_6, niacinamide, choline and pantothenic acid. Volunteers deficient in pantothenic acid were found to have reduced hydrochloric acid secretion as well as a decrease in digestive enzymes, other digestive secretions and gastric motility. It required three weeks of high potency treatment with this vitamin before normal secretions and motility were restored. Vitamin C absorption is more efficient in the presence of hydrochloric acid presumably because it keeps ascorbic acid in the free form.

Achlorhydria

A complete lack of stomach hydrochloric acid known as achlorhydria is a feature of several diseases. The most common is chronic gastritis where the parietal cells have been destroyed by atrophy of the gastric mucosa. Cancer of the stomach is usually characterized by achlorhydria, mainly because the tumour envelops the parietal cells so they no longer function. One of the diagnostic features of pernicious anaemia is finding that there is no hydrochloric acid produced. Even when the anaemia responds to vitamin B_{12} injections, there is no effect upon the gastric mucosa and hydrochloric acid secretion is still curtailed. When the stomach is partially or fully removed by surgery, the source of hydrochloric acid disappears so that digestion can only start in the mildly alkaline conditions of the small intestine. In these circumstances and indeed in any other condition where achlorhydria is a feature the consequence is the same. There is an increased chance of cancer in the gastro-intestinal tract. We shall now examine why this is so, and look at the best way to combat it.

One of the more potent group of carcinogens, i.e. cancer producing agents, is the nitrosamines. They are substances known to be associated with increased incidence of cancers of the bladder, the oesophagus and the stomach. Sources of nitrosamines include cigarettes, chewing tobacco and snuff. Even non-smokers are exposed to them by way of sidestream smoke from cigarettes. Betel-nuts contain nitrosamines and as the nuts are chewed, the carcinogens are swallowed and enter the stomach and small intestine. Low levels of nitrosamines are present in cured meat products and malt beverages.

It is not only foods that provide us with nitrosamines. Cosmetics, corrosion inhibitors and a wide variety of rubber products have been found to contain ready-made nitrosamines. Even some rubber teats for baby bottles have been found to be contaminated with these substances.

Nitrosamines can also be formed in the stomach by the interaction of two other food constituents, namely, amines and nitrites. Nitrites are readily formed from nitrates, found, for example, in many vegetables and in drinking water and they are also added to cured meats, bacon, sausages and the like. Nitrites are excellent preservatives which is why they are added to foods.

Amines are natural constituents of foods (for example the characteristic smell of fish is due to them) but are also widely used in cosmetics and drugs. Neither amines nor nitrites are likely to cause cancer on their own but when they react together, the result is the carcinogenic nitrosamines. However, what has emerged from recent research is the fact that nitrosamines are more likely to be formed in a stomach that lacks hydrochloric acid. Once the nitrosamine has been formed it can then act anywhere within the digestive tract or be absorbed and produce its carcinogenic effect elsewhere.

Hence the simplest way to prevent nitrosamine formation is to inactivate the nitrites or the amines. The most effective agents for this are vitamins C and E which harmlessly detoxify nitrites. With these out of the way, there is no chance of nitrosamine formation. At the same time there is evidence appearing that vitamins C and E can also combine with and render harmless the preformed nitrosamines.

It would appear then that an adequate intake of vitamins C and E daily is the best protection against nitrosamines but it is of even more importance if the stomach has ceased producing hydrochloric acid. For complete effectiveness these vitamins must be taken with food, preferably 100 mg of each. If we wish to take hydrochloric acid by mouth what is the best way? It is possible to drink hydrochloric acid in a very diluted form but the practice is not recommended for self-treatment. It is likely to cause damage to the teeth, and heartburn. Usually it is introduced straight into the stomach via a tube so this is a technique reserved for the medical practitioner. There is also doubt as to the efficiency of hydrochloric acid administered in this way. A more useful supplement is to introduce hydrochloric acid in combined, solid form. Betaine hydrochloride is a white powder that can be produced in tablet form. Once dissolved this material yields 25 per cent of its weight as hydrochloric acid. The usual dose is between 60 and 500 mg of betaine hydrochloride taken just after meals. Glutamic acid hydrochloride acts in a similar manner but in solution it yields only 20 per cent of its weight as hydrochloric acid. For this reason the recommended intake is 0.6 to 1.8 g during meals.

There is no doubt that hydrochloric acid is an important secretory agent of the stomach but like so many other body constituents it is most effective when carefully controlled. Some people will go through life happily unaware of any deviation from the normal state of affairs. For those of the emotional type and who undergo periods of stress there must be an awareness of what excessive hydrochloric acid can do. It is more sensible for them to carry around nuts, dried fruit, protein wafers, malted milk tablets and the like, to counteract any hyperacidity, rather than alkali tablets. At the other end of the scale, once achlorhydria has been established, hydrochloric acid tablets and, more importantly, vitamins C and E should form part of their everyday supplementation.

5

The Role of Infection in Peptic Ulcers

At the turn of the twentieth century some doctors proposed that gastritis and peptic ulcers might be due to a bacterial infection. However, since no harmful bacteria could be isolated from the stomach in those suffering from these complaints, the idea of infection being a cause was dropped. Recent studies, however, have confirmed that bacterial infection plays an important role in the development of peptic ulcers.

In 1975 in Southampton, Howard Steer published pictures taken with an electron microscope of spiral bacteria related to gastritis. Conventional methods to cultivate these bacteria in the laboratory, a prerequisite for further study, failed and interest in the bacteria waned. Fortunately, Drs Robin Warren and Barry Marshall at the Royal Perth Hospital in Western Australia persevered with attempts to culture the bacteria; by a happy chance, thanks to a bank holiday weekend, one culture was left to incubate for a more prolonged period and grew profusely. This was in April 1982 and the bacterium was given the name *Campylobacter pyloridis*. The association of this microorganization with peptic ulcer was confirmed in 1985 by Dr Marshall in 114 infected patients at Fremantle Hospital, Australia. The bacteria were identified by the original Royal Perth Hospital team as a new genus, given the new name *Helicobacter pylori* in 1989. The discovery of H. pyloria has revolutionized the therapy of gastric and duodenal ulcers using both medical and natural methods.

The Prevalence of H. Pylori Infection

H. pylori is one of the most common chronic infections, responsible for almost all cases of chronic gastritis which heals when the infection is eradicated. This organism is very strongly associated with duodenal ulcer and also has associations with gastric ulcer and with gastric cancer. In addition, the bacterium affects the secretory function of the stomach; its discovery has revolutionized our knowledge of the causes and treatment of peptic ulcers and even gastric cancer. Only in cases of ulceration induced by the non-steroidal anti-inflammatory drugs used to treat arthritis does H. pylori appear to play no part.

The stomach of practically all those with duodenal ulcer (with the above-mentioned exception) is colonized by H. pylori, yet the number of infected individuals in any community greatly exceeds those who go on to develop a duodenal ulcer. Why most of us have this infection yet only 10 per cent of us develop ulcers is not yet understood, but it is possible that some strains of H. pylori are more virulent than others. In Western countries the prevalence of H. pylori increases with age from about 20 per cent at 20 years to over 50 per cent at 50 years. In developing countries this prevalence is much higher, often reaching 80 per cent by the age of 5 years, which may reflect poorer hygienic approaches in such communities. Some of these factors also correlate with the incidence of gastric cancer. There is no evidence that H. pylori itself is cancer-forming, but the bacterium leads to gastric degeneration, which can in turn lead to chronic gastritis.

How H. Pylori May Function

H. pylori is likely to spread through the oral/faecal route. Infection usually starts in early childhood. A healthy immune system may resist it but it is a very tough bacterium and, once acquired, difficult to get rid of. Once established in the stomach and start of the duodenum it can damage the mucosal layer by causing inflammation, so giving rise to gastritis and duodenitis. This makes the mucosal layers particularly susceptible to attack by aggressive factors such as acid, pepsin, bile and drugs, all of which can cause ulceration. The bacterium also has a direct effect on the secretory function of the stomach by stimulating the increased release of gastrin, which in turn causes increased secretion of gastric acid. This damaging effect of H. pylori was confirmed when it was shown that, in those suffering with duodenal ulcer, six times more acid is released into the stomach when the bacterium is present than when it is not. The reason for this massive increase is not clear, but what is known is that once H. pylori has been eradicated, gastric acid secretion reverts to normal. A parallel situation occurs when pepsin secretion is measured: this too reverts to normal once the bacterium has been removed. The end result is that colonization with H. pylori causes hyperacidity which in turn favours abnormal changes in the gastric mucosa (lining of the stomach), opening the way for serious damage of this layer and eventually ulcer formation.

The Effect of H. Pylori in Peptic Ulcers

Duodenal ulcer is virtually unknown in H. pylori-negative individuals, so we can assume that the organism must make a major contribution to the causation of the disease and in maintaining it. However, there must also be other factors contributing to the development of the ulcer since it can be healed by giving acid-suppressing drugs which have no effect on H. pylori. On the other hand, eradication of H. pylori alone can heal an ulcer without any other therapy. What is significant is the observation that the chances of recurrence of ulcers are decreased dramatically, no matter which course of therapy is followed, if H. pylori is eradicated. The biggest problem with drug therapy for duodenal ulcers is the high incidence of recurrence after the ulcer has healed – such relapses do not occur if the bacterium is removed. This observation would suggest that eradication of the infective agent appears to change the natural history of duodenal ulcer. Nevertheless, even in the absence of infection, exposure to all the other risk factors may cause recurrence of the ulcer, so steps must be taken to control these also.

The association between gastric ulcer and H. pylori is less strong than with duodenal ulcer, since only about 80 per cent of patients suffering from gastric ulcer are infected with H. pylori. There have been fewer studies on the effect of eradication of the organism on the healing of gastric ulcers, but evidence available suggests that getting rid of the H. pylori decreases the chances of recurrence of these types of ulcer also.

Eradication of H. Pylori

Removing H. pylori from the lining of the stomach is difficult because it thrives on the surface of the mucosa but beneath the protective layer of mucus. It can survive in the deep gastric pits because antibacterial agents cannot reach into these recesses from which the bacterium can emerge later to reinfect the stomach lining. Regrettably, it has also been observed that H. pylori can readily develop resistance to the available antibiotics. It has been calculated that resistant strains are present in about 20 per cent of women in the West and in 80 per cent of women in developing countries. For this reason modern therapy against peptic ulcers is moving away from treatment with one agent only and is now tending towards using two or more agents simultaneously.

There is as yet no definitive treatment regimen for H. pylori infection. Many different combinations of antimicrobial agents, given in varying doses and for different periods of time have been tried, but no firm conclusion can be drawn as to the best. The most effective single therapy at present is that of bismuth, since H. pylori does not develop a resistance to it and it results in a lower relapse rate than any other single treatment – however even bismuth is still less effective than the combined use of two or more agents (polytherapy).

Failure of procedures to eradicate H. pylori can be attributed to three main reasons: resistance to the drugs, poor compliance on the part of patients due to the increased risk, since a number of drugs are involved, of side-effects (in up to 35 per cent of patients), and the inability of patients to stick to complicated drug schedules. Despite these disadvantages triple therapies are showing great promise – with eradication rates ranging from 70 to 80 per cent.

Who Will Benefit?

There is distinct disagreement amongst gastroenterologists about the role of H. pylori eradication. Some advocate this approach for all H. pylori-positive ulcer patients, whilst others reserve the therapy for those in relapse after conventional medical therapy. Others restrict eradication just to those with complications of ulcer disease. Most workers in the H. pylori area advise eradication therapy immediately the infection is diagnosed. The only exception is in those people who have developed peptic ulcers as a result of treatment with anti-arthritic drugs. Some people, of course, will not respond to H. pylori eradication, and because of the growing public awareness of the relationship between the organism and gastric cancer such people are likely to seek reassurances from their doctor. Treatment by other methods then becomes of paramount

importance. Only complete healing of the ulcer combined with total eradication of H. pylori can reduce the
possibility of mucosal malignancy.

Vitamins and H. Pylori

There is an observed relationship between H. pylori
infection and levels of vitamin C in the stomach.
Those who are infected with the bacterium have lowered levels of the active antioxidant form of vitamin C
in their gastric juice. This abnormality is readily
reversed by successful antibiotic therapy to eradicate
the infective agent. Effects of other antioxidant vitamins on H. pylori were observed only in animals,
where vitamin E was found to protect the lining of the
stomach against injury. Recently, however, studies on
human beings at the Northwick Park Institute for
Medical Research in Harrow have confirmed the
important role of vitamin E in controlling H. pylori
infection. In the patients studied, vitamin E levels
were increased in two areas of the stomach: the main
body (or corpus) and the area adjacent to the duodenum (or antrum).

Normal, healthy individuals had higher levels of
vitamin E in the main body of the stomach than in the
area adjacent to the duodenum. The reverse situation
was found in those patients with H. pylori infection:
they had diminished levels of vitamin E in the main

body of the stomach but normal levels in the duodenal end, where most ulcers occur. The authors of the study concluded that vitamin E was mobilized from the corpus of the stomach to the antrum when this became infected with H. pylori.

It is, therefore, imperative to maintain high levels of both vitamins C and E in the stomach to reduce the chances of peptic ulceration. However, whilst these vitamins are both effective antioxidants and hence prime stimulators of the body's immune system, it must be remembered that other vitamins and trace minerals are also important in this respect. These include beta-carotene, folic acid, riboflavin (vitamin B_2), zinc, selenium and vitamin A. All of the antioxidant nutrients are needed for an efficient immune system, which in turn will ensure the body's best defence against bacterial infections such as Helicobacter pylori. At the same time, these antioxidant nutrients appear to confer protection against some cancers, and it is possible that adequate intakes of all of them will prevent peptic ulceration from progressing to a malignant growth in the stomach.

6

Medical Treatments of Peptic Ulcers

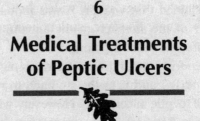

The aims of medical and medicinal treatment in duodenal and gastric ulcers are the relief of symptoms, the healing of the ulcer crater, the prevention of recurrence and the prevention of complications. We have seen that successful eradication of H. pylori heals ulcers and, perhaps more importantly, lowers the relapse rate of duodenal ulcer and probably also of gastric ulcer.

Anticholinergics

These drugs are given to delay emptying of the stomach, which can be rapid in the case of uncomplicated duodenal ulcer. In this way antacid-retention is prolonged; when taken in adequate doses, anticholinergics also diminish acid secretion. These drugs are most effective at night when regular hourly intake of antacids is impractical. Tincture of belladonna, which is in this class of drugs, is still widely used.

Like all drugs, however, anticholinergics provide their share of side-effects. Dry mouth or blurred vision (or both) are not uncommon. Less common but more serious are urinary retention and glaucoma. Complete pyloric obstruction may develop in those who previously suffered only partial obstruction. Anyone with oesophagitis or oesophageal ulcers cannot take anticholinergic drugs because of potential side-effects. For the same reason, smokers should abstain whilst on these drugs.

Modern thinking queries the effectiveness of anticholinergic drugs in the short- or long-term healing of either gastric or duodenal ulcer because of a lack of controlled trials. As well as being contraindicated in glaucoma, they should not be used in patients with heartburn because, by lowering oesophageal sphincter pressure, they might make this condition worse. One ray of hope in this class of drugs is the recent introduction of pirenzepine, which has a mild antisecretory activity. Controlled clinical trials indicate that this drug does speed the healing of duodenal ulcer.

Combined Therapy with Anticholinergics

Some gastro-enterologists advocate administering anticholinergics with another therapy, such as antacids, where the slowing down of gastric emptying might increase the length of time during which the antacid can get to work on neutralizing stomach acids. Similarly, giving anticholinergics together with acid-suppressing drugs has been advocated by other specialists in the field, but their claims of efficacy have not been confirmed by others. There is no hard evidence that anticholinergics combined with other drugs are any better than anticholinergics alone in treating peptic ulcer – and of course, combining drugs introduces extra chances of side-effects.

Sucralfate

Sucralfate is a combination of aluminium with a sugar derivative. When it comes into contact with gastric acid it becomes very viscous and forms a protective coating on the damaged stomach lining. Although sucralfate does not inhibit acid secretion it can absorb pepsin and bile salts, both factors in peptic ulceration. In controlled clinical trials, sucralfate was shown to be effective in accelerating the healing rate of duodenal ulcers. It is generally regarded as a safe drug but it can interact with other medicines. There is also a danger that the aluminium present will be absorbed. Constipation is the most likely side-effect.

Drugs that Reduce Acid Secretion

Most physicians now use therapeutic agents called histamine H_2 receptor blocking agents for treating peptic ulcers. These drugs act specifically by inhibiting the secretion of stomach acid. Usually the H_2 receptors in the stomach react to naturally-produced histamine by stimulating the production and secretion of hydrochloric acid. Hence, by blocking these H_2 receptors in a specific manner, they no longer function and acid secretion stops.

The three most commonly used drugs are ranitidine, cimetidine and famotidine. They are usually taken with each meal and at bedtime. Gastric acidity is lowered and healing of the gastric and duodenal ulcers is promoted. Whilst symptoms are commonly relieved within the first week, complete healing of the ulcer may take between two and eight weeks. The usual length of treatment is four weeks. Not all ulcers are healed by these measures, but the healing rate increases with length of treatment perhaps up to 12 weeks. Unfortunately, the longer the therapy lasts the more chances there are of side-effects.

Self-therapy:

All three of these drugs can now be purchased without prescription from pharmacies. However, the potencies of the drugs sold in this way are below those prescribed by a doctor. These low potencies are not suitable for treating peptic ulcers and should only be used by an individual for relief from the symptoms of indigestion, heartburn and excess acid. No more than two tablets should be taken in any 24-hour period. Relief from symptoms usually lasts about nine hours after taking one tablet of any of the preparations. The weight of active ingredient in each of the preparations varies because each of the three substances is different in its activity. However, one tablet of either ranitidine, cimetidine or famotidine will provide the equivalent amount of acid-suppressing activity.

What Are the Side-effects?:

Diarrhoea, muscle pain, dizziness and skin rash may occasionally occur with all three drugs. The most common adverse effect of cimetidine is mild sedation and tiredness, which disappear once the drug is withdrawn. These side-effects are not usually severe enough to warrant cessation of treatment. More serious are impotence, lack of sperm in semen and other effects induced by the anti-sex hormone effects of cimetidine (and unique to this drug). Fortunately, such effects are rare. In addition, cases of acute pancreatitis and nephritis (inflammation of the kidneys) have been associated with cimetidine.

Acid-suppressive Drugs and Cancer:

One of the more serious controversies concerning cimetidine therapy was centred on the possibility of the drug causing gastric cancer. Out of 9,504 patients who had taken cimetidine, gastric cancer was diagnosed in 74. Twenty-three were diagnosed before treatment had started; 29 had gastric cancer within six months of starting therapy. Only 8 patients out of 8,994 controls (who did not receive the drug) developed gastric cancer over the same (one-year) period. It is possible that cimetidine had been used unwittingly to treat gastric cancer (which had been there all the time) according to those reporting the trials.[1]

These observations were made when cimetidine was the only acid-suppressive drug available, but concern has been expressed about possible cancer-inducing effects of long-term treatment with all gastric-acid anti-secretory drugs. Inhibition of stomach acid favours bacterial colonization of the stomach. Enzymes produced by these bacteria can catalyse the conversion of dietary nitrates to nitrites, with subsequent formation of carcinogenic nitrosamines. Hence it is not by direct action of the drugs that there is a possibility of cancer, but rather that the *lack* of acid may stimulate the growth of harmful bacteria, probably Helicobacter pylori. Eradication of this bacterium may therefore help to prevent stomach cancer. The best natural protectant is vitamin C, which prevents formation of the harmful nitrosamines. Although vitamin C is a weak acid, unlike gastric acid it will not form or exacerbate ulcers and so it can be taken in perfect safety. However, at present there are no grounds for withholding long-term H_2-blockade.

Possible Recurrence of Ulcers:

Having established that H_2 antagonists will heal peptic ulcers in most patients, the question remains on how to prevent their recurrence. When treatment with these drugs is stopped after ulcer healing, up to 80 per cent of patients will have ulcer recurrence within one year. For this reason, the patient is often put onto maintenance therapy at a lower dose. Despite this, experience in the UK has indicated a remission rate of 30 per cent in the case of duodenal ulcers and that of 20 per cent in gastric ulcers in the first 12 months of maintenance therapy. There are, however, unexplained differences between patients in various countries. In duodenal ulcers, recurrence during one year maintenance on ranitidine was 26 per cent in the UK, 16 per cent in Germany and a massive 60 per cent in Austria and Belgium.

There are no obvious reasons for these variations. Age, sex, smoking habits and drug tolerance appeared to play no part. What was apparent, however, was that when maintenance therapy was discontinued after one year, relapses occurred at the same rate as before treatment. The conclusion reached was that drug therapy with H_2 receptor antagonists merely suppresses the disease and does not alter its natural history.

In 1982 a World Congress of Gastroenterology, held in Stockholm, assessed the efficiency of these drugs. Whilst there was no doubt of their usefulness in healing ulcers, no clear-cut decision was reached on how to prevent their recurrence in chronic disease. The choice lay between long-term maintenance therapy, with the risk of side-effects, and surgery.

One speaker suggested there were signs that the natural history of gastric and duodenal ulcers in the UK was changing to a 'less aggressive' form. Fewer patients were being presented for emergency surgery because of perforation or haemorrhage. This trend had actually started before the H_2 antagonist drugs had been introduced, so there was some other, less obvious reason.

Unhappily, though, it was reported that the total incidence of ulcer disease is not falling and the sad conclusion was that more and more patients would end up on long-term drug therapy. No one suggested that dietary principles could be the best cure for and preventative of peptic ulcers.

The most promising approach to preventing the recurrence of peptic ulcers is, as we have seen, the eradication of Helicobacter pylori. Whilst it is as yet too soon to reach definite conclusions about this approach since it is a relatively recent one, the signs are promising. The fact remains, however, that many people appear to go through life with H. pylori in their stomachs yet never suffering gastro-intestinal problems. There are many questions yet to be answered.

Proton Pump Inhibitors:

We have seen that the parietal cells of the stomach are responsible for the production of gastric acid. The manner in which this is achieved is by a proton 'pump'. The pump consists of an enzyme that provides energy for the secretion of protons (that is, positively-charged hydrogen atoms) which confer acidity on the gastric acids. The higher the concentration of protons, the stronger the acid. Hence any drug that inhibits the proton pump will reduce the secretion of stomach acid. The first successful drug with this property is omeprazole (trade name Losec); later variations include lansoprazole and pantoprazole.

These drugs are readily destroyed by gastric acid, so for oral use the tablets are coated with a special finish that protects the contents until they are beyond the stomach. Of course, once they start functioning the acid is no longer present to denature them, so their activity increases. At the peak of their activity they will suppress acid production for 24 hours with a single dose. A one-a-day dosage regime is attractive for any therapy, and when taken in the morning a tablet will suppress acidity in the stomach for a whole day. This is one reason why many doctors are switching from the H_2 receptor antagonists to omeprazole and similar drugs.

Whilst treatment with omeprazole generally is extremely well tolerated, like any drug it can cause side-effects. These include diarrhoea, skin rashes and headache. Very rarely such side-effects are sufficient to warrant cessation of treatment. Mild mental confusion in severely ill patients has occasionally been reported. However, one major concern is the drug's ability to cause a very large decrease in gastric acidity, which leads in turn to increased susceptibility to stomach infection, exacerbation of existing infection, and rises in gastrin concentration. All of these factors predispose to potential gastric cancer, although there has not yet been any confirmation of this in humans. Very long-term treatment with omeprazole, which is unusual, is more likely (at least in theory) to give rise to these problems. Most consultant gastric physicians are now tending to prescribe antibiotics to eradicate H. pylori along with omeprazole to prevent potential problems.

Prostaglandins:

A third approach to suppression of gastric acid is the use of a synthetic prostaglandin called misoprostol.

Prostaglandins are a class of substances which have hormone-like activity and are produced usually by the body itself. The starting material for natural body synthesis of prostaglandins is the polyunsaturated fatty acids in the diet. Whilst misoprostol has a milder acid-suppression function than the other two types of drugs discussed above, it does tend to enhance the stomach lining's defences against acid. As prostaglandins are very potent substances, misoprostol tends to be prescribed in microgram (one millionth of one gram) doses which leave little room for error. Also, because they act like hormones, prostaglandins are readily destroyed by body processes and so must be given at regular intervals over a day.

Typical side-effects of misoprostol include abdominal pain or diarrhoea, usually within the first few days of therapy. The drug can induce abortion so it is contraindicated in pregnancy and in women of child-bearing age who may be likely to conceive during the treatment period.

Misoprostol has not found a place in the routine treatment of duodenal or gastric ulcer because of unimpressive healing rates and unwanted side-effects. Its main application is as a preventative therapy in those receiving long-term anti-arthritic drugs, as it protects against the possibility of these drugs causing a gastric or duodenal ulcer. When such ulcers are the result of therapy with anti-arthritic preparations, misoprostol can help to heal them and is sometimes used instead of H_2-blockers.

Preparations Containing Liquorice

Liquorice has a soothing (or demulcent) action on the mucous membranes, which is why it is used to relieve coughs and sore throats. It also has an expectorant action which helps to remove the phlegm that is often the cause of throat irritation. This demulcent property is the reason why liquorice is also a traditional remedy for peptic ulceration.

Liquorice has mild anti-inflammatory properties but in addition can act like the corticosteroid hormones produced in the adrenal glands. The latter are undesirable, so the ideal preparation of liquorice for treating ulcers would be one that retains the demulcent and anti-inflammatory properties but reduces the hormone-like activity. Such a preparation is deglycyrrhizinized liquorice, which has been found to be of great use in healing peptic ulcers. (For more about using liquorice to promote natural healing, see page 118.)

Another approach is to modify chemically a constituent of liquorice to produce an anti-ulcer drug. This is called carbenoxolone. Like all liquorice preparations it functions by reducing the inflammation (in this case around the ulcer) and by causing the secretion of large amounts of thick protective mucus (which cover the ulcer). Thus by preventing contact of hydrochloric acid with the ulcer, the mucus allows natural healing to take place. At the same time liquorice preparations stimulate cell regeneration, which accelerates the rate of healing.

Because liquorice and its derivatives still retain adrenal cortex hormone-like activities, they can have an effect upon the minerals of the body. This leads to sodium and water retention, causing oedema. At the same time there is excessive loss of potassium in the urine, along with excessive alkaline conditions in the body. High blood-pressure has been reported as well as a mild, reversible, diabetic-like condition. Heartburn can follow the ingestion of carbenoxolone in tablet form.

Liquorice and its derivatives can therefore be regarded as successful in the treatment of gastric and duodenal ulcers, but their use must be tempered with caution. In moderate amounts the root can have a positive beneficial effect, but at the same time its possible side-effects must be monitored since they can be detrimental. Deglycyrrhizinized liquorice appears to be the preparation of choice in terms of safety and efficacy.

Treating Stress with Drugs

It is well established that rest and removal from stressful circumstances at home or in the workplace will act as a useful ally to the treatment of peptic ulcer. At one time admission to hospital was virtually mandatory in those with peptic ulcer but this practice is now reserved only for extreme cases where complications have arisen. However, in attempts to relieve stress some doctors have prescribed mild tranquillizers and sedatives to their peptic ulcer patients. Such indiscriminate prescribing is now recognized as highly undesirable and is not regarded as good practice. Discussion of the particular life circumstance and lifestyle with the patient is often more helpful and productive in achieving better symptom control. There is some evidence that some kinds of anti-depressive drugs may accelerate the healing of duodenal ulcers, although the rate of recurrence is not affected. However, the evidence is considered insufficient to suggest these anti-depressants as a routine therapy in treating duodenal ulcer. When depression co-exists with peptic ulcer disease, each condition should be treated separately. There is no indication as to how anti-depressants may act in alleviating the symptoms of peptic ulcer.

Surgical Treatment of Peptic Ulcers

With the advent of acid-suppressing drugs, surgical treatment of peptic ulcers has now become the exception rather than the rule. Nevertheless there remain in the population many individuals who have had peptic ulcer surgery in the 1950s–1970s, up to half of whom will experience some long-term side-effects of their operation. Surgery is still performed in peptic ulcer where prolonged medical treatment has failed, for bleeding and perforation, for pyloric stenosis and where there is a suspicion of malignancy in gastric ulcer. In addition, surgery may be the only option for those who live in remote areas with limited access to medical facilities and in occupations where a sudden gastric bleeding or perforation may endanger the lives of others.

Types of Operation:

Uncomplicated duodenal ulcer is now invariably treated by some variant of vagotomy. Vagotomy is the cutting of the vagus nerve to the stomach. The vagus is the main nerve controlling gastric function and, by careful selection of the site of severance, it is possible to reduce acid secretion without affecting other functions. Sometimes part of the stomach is removed or resected, an operation called partial gastrectomy; sometimes this is combined with vagotomy. Complete gastrectomy – that is, removal of the whole stomach, is usually reserved for gastric cancer.

Consequences of Gastric Surgery:

The major problems following gastric surgery are:

Early Dumping

This is common and is characterized by a feeling of fullness and abdominal distension within 30 minutes of starting a meal. It is usually accompanied by nausea, vomiting, sweating, faintness and palpitations. These symptoms are the result of accelerated gastric emptying, a consequence of partial gastrectomy. Treatment is dietary. This means cutting out sugary foods, including milk. Carbohydrates should be taken as starchy foods in small, frequent meals. Soluble dietary fibre such as pectin may be helpful in slowing gastric emptying. It is sometimes useful for sufferers to lie down for half an hour immediately after eating.

Bile Vomiting

This is associated with partial gastrectomy and is due to reflux into the stomach of bile-containing duodenal contents. These disrupt the mucus layer protecting the stomach lining. There is no proven dietary advice for this symptom although antacids may help, as will substances that bind like acids (such as cholestyramine). Strangely, drugs that accelerate gastric emptying may relieve the condition and these are often prescribed.

Diarrhoea

This is a frequent complaint after gastric surgery but is most common after vagotomy. It is due to a failure to control gastric emptying and interruption of the nerve supply to the small bowel. The result is rapid passage of food through the gut, increased bile acids in the colon and mild malabsorption. The dietary treatment is similar to that for early dumping and an anti-diarrhoeal such as codeine or loperamide may be taken or prescribed.

Late Dumping

This condition is rare and is characterized by sweating, palpitations, weakness, confusion and occasionally loss of consciousness 2–3 hours after a meal. The symptoms are those of hypoglycaemia. Management of an acute attack is to take sugar or glucose by mouth. The long-term approach is that recommended for hypoglycaemia. Prevention requires the early dumping diet regimen.

Total Gastrectomy:

Total removal of the stomach is still performed, albeit occasionally, but the consequences can be severe. Eating almost always causes abdominal discomfort, fullness and nausea and there may be dumping and bile vomiting. Malnutrition is common and supportive dietary management is essential. Meals must be small and frequent, say every 2 hours, and must not contain high levels of sugar and milk. Food must be chewed thoroughly, and indigestible food avoided.

Dietary supplements of all vitamins and minerals are mandatory, with particular reference to iron and vitamin B_{12}.

Nutritional Consequences of Gastric Surgery:

Weight loss, iron-deficiency anaemia, vitamin B_{12} deficiency and osteomalacia (softening of the bone due to deficiency of vitamin D and calcium) may all occur after gastric surgery. Weight loss is directly related to a reduced food intake, but malabsorption plays no significant part. Dietary measures must be undertaken to maintain body weight within the normal range for the individual.

Anaemia is usually of the iron-deficient type and is due to a combination of reduced iron intake, poor absorption of food iron and increased losses from the stomach and intestines because of inflammation and occasional ulceration. A liquid iron preparation is the preferred supplementary treatment. A reduced mechanism for absorbing vitamin B_{12} after gastric surgery may give rise to the particular anaemia associated with a lack of the vitamin after a prolonged time; the gastro-intestinal system may have to be by-passed with intramuscular injections of the vitamin.

Osteomalacia and osteoporosis (honeycombing of the bones) are more common in those who have undergone gastric surgery. In the younger patient, supplementation with vitamin D and calcium can help to strengthen the bones. In the older male and female patient similar supplementation is essential – but in addition the older female may require Hormone Replacement Therapy (HRT) to control the osteoporosis. There are non-hormonal drugs which perform a similar function in older males. The two conditions do not normally appear until 6–10 years after gastric surgery, but supplementary regimes should be undertaken as soon as possible after the operation and exercise must be maintained in all groups.

1. MOLLER, H. et al. Use of Cimetidine and other peptic ulcer drugs in Denmark 1977–1990 with analysis of the risk of gastric cancer among Cimetidine users. GUT 1992;33:1166–9.

7

Natural Treatments of Peptic Ulcers

There is published evidence in the medical and scientific literature that peptic ulcers will often respond to natural treatments without the use of synthetic drugs. We shall now examine the efficacy of these natural measures, which include vitamins, minerals, herbs, vegetables and their extracts.

Diet

Diet looms very large in the self-therapy of most patients with peptic ulcer. Almost all will avoid fatty, fried, spicy and rich meals because they become aware that such foods will produce pain and distension. Each individual will also discover other foods that upset them and will therefore tend to avoid eating them. The older traditional treatments for peptic ulcer such as bland diets were never proved to be effective and are no longer regarded as essential. Milk was central to these diets, but its neutralizing activity is only brief and the stomach responds by producing even more acid. There is some evidence that frequent, small meals help because food is a powerful neutralizer of stomach acid. The simplest philosophy to follow for the peptic ulcer sufferer is 'avoid what upsets you, eat little and often and go to bed with an empty stomach.' (For more about dietary approaches to peptic ulcer, see Chapter 8.)

Deglycyrrhizinated Liquorice

Liquorice root has been a traditional herbal medicine for peptic ulcers for at least 200 years, but in the whole, raw state it was found to cause severe side-effects when taken at high potency over a prolonged period. Reports have appeared in the medical literature over the last 30 years that excessive ingestion of liquorice as confectionery, soft drinks, medicines or chewing tobacco have caused adverse effects. These include excessive loss of potassium leading to low blood levels of this mineral, high blood-pressure, congestive heart failure and cardiac arrest. Also noted were headache, muscle weakness, muscle wasting, paralysis and menstrual problems. The main toxic component causing these effects is glycyrrhetinic acid; this is believed to act like a potent corticosteroid since these too cause similar adverse effects. The first symptoms of excess liquorice is retention of water. It must be stressed that such effects are associated only with very large intakes of liquorice usually taken over long periods. Moderate amounts of the root will not give rise to such problems.

Fortunately it is a simple procedure to remove the glycyrrhetinic acid from liquorice; the resulting product, whilst effective against peptic ulcers, does not produce the side-effects noted above.

In controlled studies deglycyrrhizinated liquorice (DGL) has been shown to be at least as effective as the newest class of anti-ulcer drugs (the H_2-receptor blocking agents) in accelerating the healing of gastric and duodenal ulcers. DGL also appears to protect against aspirin-induced damage to the stomach lining. The herb provides regeneration of the ulcerated lining by increasing the number of mucus-secreting glands as well as the number of mucus-secreting cells in each gland. The resulting excess mucus then acts as a protective barrier against stomach acid, allowing normal healing processes to take place. DGL is available as CAVED-S and can be bought without prescription.

The Use of Cabbage Juice

Professor Garnet Cheney, of the Stanford Medical School, California, has had success with cabbage juice in the treatment of stomach ulcers. He says that it is the vitamin C factor in the juice which has such powerful healing qualities. This may be only partly true, since the same researcher reported a unique factor, called vitamin U, in cabbage leaves and other vegetables. This has been called the anti-ulcer vitamin. Vitamin U has been isolated from cabbage leaves and has also been produced by chemical synthesis. It has the chemical name (3-amino-3-carboxypropyl) dimethyl sulphonium chloride, or MMSC. It has been known under the trade names Caboagin-U, Epadyn-U, Vitas-U and Ardesyl. It is a very safe substance when consumed orally.

In a typical trial, a group of 26 people with peptic ulcers received concentrated cabbage juice (5 glasses daily) for 3 weeks. At the end of this period, 92 per cent showed evidence of healing compared with only 32 per cent of a group of 19 similar people with untreated peptic ulcers. It is of interest to note that cabbage juice is also a rich source of glutamine, an amino acid which may also have beneficial effects in treating peptic ulcers. Fortunately, cabbage juice has quite an acceptable taste since up to 1 litre daily may need to be taken when treating an ulcer.

Garlic

Oil of garlic has remarkable healing properties and has been used in Europe and Asia for centuries. Garlic is a cleanser and kills unfriendly bacteria in the large intestine, thereby lightening the duties of the liver and spleen. Garlic improves the appetite, reduces blood tension and helps to prevent thrombosis. It is excellent for respiratory troubles, is highly regarded as a nerve tonic and remedies flatulence and diarrhoea. It is recognized as a most valuable intestinal antiseptic. Garlic capsules, each containing three minims of pure oil of garlic, are readily available.

The antiseptic qualities of oil of garlic may help eradicate H. pylori; this is probably at the root of its success in healing peptic ulcers. There is evidence that deodorized garlic is effective in this manner because it contains the precursor of the active principle Allicin, called Alliin. Allicin appears to be the antiseptic substance.

Herbal Remedies

We have discussed already two herbal remedies for peptic ulcers, that is, liquorice and garlic. In addition, however, there are other traditional remedies for gastric conditions. One of the better established and more effective ones is Althaea root, otherwise known as marshmallow root. Its main active constituent is mucilage, but it also contains sterols, asparagin and lecithin, all of which contribute to its beneficial effect. Marshmallow has a demulcent action combined with an emollient or softening and soothing effect. For this reason the root is recommended for gastritis and duodenal ulcers. The usual dose is between 2 and 5 g of the dried root three times daily. A more effective preparation is a combination of marshmallow with symphytum.

Symphytum:

This is more commonly known as comfrey and is active in either the root or leafy form. Both have a demulcent action due to their content of mucilage, allantoin, symphitine and echimidine. The usual dose of dried root or dried leaves is 2–4 g or 4–8 g respectively, taken at the rate of three doses per day.

Slippery Elm Bark:

Also known as ulmus, this is another rich source of mucilage – which explains its beneficial actions as a demulcent and emollient. Unlike most herbal remedies, Slippery Elm Bark contains significant amounts of starch. The powdered bark is usually mixed with water at the rate of 1 part bark to 8 parts water. The liquid (4–16 cc) is drunk three times daily. There are, however, many commercial preparations of dried bark extract which may be more convenient to take.

Aloe vera:

This is a tropical plant whose leaves are used for medicinal purposes. A cross-section of a leaf shows the presence of a colourless gel surrounded by darker layers of pigment. The gel and the pigment have completely different medicinal properties. The pigment is a source of bitter aloes or aloin, which has a strong laxative action and is used for occasional constipation. The gel has no purgative properties and is best known for its soothing, antiseptic and healing functions. When the gel is obtained fresh from the aloe vera leaf it can be applied directly to wounds, where it helps natural healing. It has also been taken orally to treat gastric and duodenal ulcers with some success. In surgical procedures, fresh aloe vera gel has been used as an antiseptic on surgically-induced wounds and particularly on sensitive areas of the skin, for example around the eyes, when these have been damaged by burning.

Only the fresh gel has these properties. Unfortunately many of the commercial preparations available are simply an extract of the whole leaves, and so retain the purgative properties as well. There is no clinical evidence that these extracts are as safe and effective as the pure, fresh gel itself in treating peptic ulcer, although there have been anecdotal reports of success for this condition.

Vitamin A and Gastric Ulcers

There is increasing interest in using the natural food constituent vitamin A as a therapeutic agent in the treatment of gastric ulcers. It is well known that vitamin A has a protective action on the skin and mucous membranes; indeed it is one of its accepted, essential functions. For this reason it was reasoned that the vitamin had the potential for exerting a similar action against gastric ulcer. This hypothesis has been tested of vitamin A in a multi-centre, randomized, controlled trial of 60 patients with chronic gastric ulcers. The trial took place in Hungary and was reported in the *Lancet* in 1982.

There were three groups of patients. One group was treated only with antacids; the second group received similar antacids, with the addition of 150,000 iu of vitamin A daily; the third group were given the same doses of vitamin A and antacids daily, with the addition of cyproheptadine, an antihistamine drug, also daily. All patients were treated for four weeks. Ulcer sizes were measured before and after treatment in each case.

All ulcers were reduced to a significant degree, but those patients receiving vitamin A experienced a significantly greater reduction in size than those treated just with antacids. The authors concluded that 'a beneficial effect of vitamin A has been indicated in the prevention and treatment of stress ulcers in patients.'

No simple clinical trial is accepted by the medical fraternity as conclusive until it has been repeated with similar success. The above trial was conducted on patients with stress-induced gastric ulcers. It was therefore repeated on patients suffering from chronic and recurrent gastric ulcers and reported in the *International Journal of Tissue Reactions* in 1983. The second trial was a randomized, prospective study of 60 patients with chronic gastric ulcer. One group received antacids only; the second group were given antacids plus 50,000 iu vitamin A three times daily, and the third group received the same medication as the second group but with the addition of an antihistamine drug. As before, treatment was continued for four weeks. The number of patients with completely healed ulcers was higher in the groups which received vitamin A. In addition, the reduction in ulcer size was greater in patients who were given vitamin A. The authors concluded that 'vitamin A has a beneficial effect in the process of ulcer healing in patients with chronic gastric ulcer.'

One pleasing aspect of both trials was the complete lack of toxic side-effects despite the relatively high intakes of vitamin A. They suggest that 150,000 iu daily for four weeks is a dose of the vitamin easily tolerated over this period. The excellent response is an indication of natural treatment. On the other hand, as we shall see later, these results also suggest that prevention of gastric ulceration can be brought about by an adequate intake of this vitamin throughout life.

Gastric ulcers can be thought of as a pre-cancerous state, and significant correlation has been reported between body levels of vitamin A and the development of various cancers. In other words, low levels of the vitamin appear to be found regularly in cases of cancer of the lung, bladder and skin. The results of these two trials indicate a possible role for gastric protection in the efforts to keep gastric ulcer from developing into gastric cancer.

Vitamin C Deficiency and Peptic Ulcers

Established studies have indicated that the lower the levels of vitamin C in the blood, urine and stomach fluid, the greater the risk of peptic ulceration. It has also been noted that vitamin C levels are lower in those with bleeding peptic ulcers than in those with non-bleeding ones. Studies on guinea pigs, who like humans need a dietary source of vitamin C, showed that when they were fed a vitamin C-deficient diet they developed peptic ulcers.

Simple vitamin C supplementation can be an effective treatment for peptic ulcers. In a French pilot study, when the vitamin was given intravenously both gastric and duodenal ulcers healed at the same rate as that provided by other therapies. In another study, from Japan, vitamin C was used orally with ferrous sulphate; the combination was found to be effective in increasing the healing rate of gastric ulcers. For some unknown reason this treatment was not successful in healing duodenal ulcers. Whilst there is no doubt that people with even a mild deficiency of vitamin C, who also suffer from peptic ulcers, will benefit from supplementation with the vitamin, the role of vitamin C in healing ulcers in those who are not deficient is not yet clarified. However, since deficiency levels of the vitamin have not yet been defined for all areas of the body it would be a sensible precaution for anyone with peptic ulcer to ensure an adequate intake of the vitamin. A typical therapeutic approach would be 500 mg of a buffered vitamin C to be taken before every meal and at bedtime.

Vitamin E and Peptic Ulcers

Both vitamin C and vitamin E are prime protectors against damage done by free radicals to the organs and cell membranes of the body. Vitamin C is water soluble and so protects the aqueous phases (fluids in the body), and vitamin E by virtue of its fat solubility acts to protect the fatty phases of the body. Since peptic ulceration primarily attacks the cells lining the stomach and duodenum it would be expected that protecting them is the responsibility of both vitamins, but vitamin E in particular is needed by the fatty cell membranes. Body fats are particularly liable to attack by free radicals, a process akin to rancidity in fatty foods and known as lipid peroxidation. Recent studies from Russia have indicated that peptic ulcer disease may be due to both an exacerbation of lipid peroxidation and lack of the protective vitamin E. In carrying out its role of protecting against lipid peroxidation vitamin E is itself destroyed, so it must be constantly replenished from the diet to prevent deficiency.

Published studies have indicated that vitamin E supplementation protects against stomach ulcers in both animals and human beings. Russian studies have gone further and concluded that the vitamin in therapeutic doses may aid in the actual healing of ulcers of both the stomach and duodenum. A typical daily supplementary intake in this respect is 400–800 iu vitamin E. These are preliminary studies but the encouraging results warrant further examination. This amount of vitamin E is perfectly safe when taken over the short period of treatment for peptic ulcer.

Mineral Supplementation

Minerals are used as antacids in the treatment of peptic ulcers.

Sodium bicarbonate and calcium carbonate (chalk) are the most potent antacids, but they are absorbed, resulting in high levels of sodium and calcium minerals in the body. The result is a condition called alkalosis or milk-alkali syndrome. Symptoms include nausea, weakness and headache – leading, after chronic indigestion, to kidney damage. Hence soluble antacids must be used with particular caution in those whose ulcer symptoms include vomiting and haemorrhage. Those who are dehydrated because of these conditions or who suffer from high blood-pressure or kidney trouble should not take absorbable antacids. Blood calcium levels may also rise, leading to calcification in the soft tissues and organs of the body.

The most commonly used non-absorbable antacids are aluminium hydroxide, magnesium hydroxide and magnesium carbonate. Aluminium hydroxide is regarded as relatively safe, yet the following side-effects may occur. Phosphate depletion can result from the binding of phosphate by aluminium in the gastro-intestinal tract. As a result, blood phosphate levels fall; the body then extracts more from the bone to make up the deficit, so the bones weaken. The result is weakness, malaise and loss of appetite. Eventually the bone becomes so demineralized that breakages occur relatively easily. Such potential problems are, however, unlikely in practice since our Western diet tends to provide far more phosphorus than is needed as an essential mineral. As long as these antacids are not taken regularly over many months, preventing the absorption of phosphorus to a significant degree is not likely to be a problem.

Aluminium hydroxide may also cause constipation. Although alleged to be totally insoluble it is possible that some of the aluminium will dissolve and be absorbed. At high levels this mineral can be quite toxic. Fears that long-term use of aluminium hydroxide gel may promote the development of Alzheimer's disease appear to be unfounded. Despite the insolubility of the mineral there have been claims of significant absorption of the aluminium into the bloodstream, but these have never been proven.

Magnesium hydroxide makes an effective antacid. It can cause diarrhoea, so is often given with aluminium hydroxide to prevent the constipation induced by the latter. This is fine if the amount taken is carefully controlled. As some magnesium is certainly absorbed, this treatment is not suitable for those suffering from kidney problems.

In modern treatments, aluminium-magnesium antacids are usually preferred to those containing sodium bicarbonate because of the latter's high sodium content, short duration of action and possible alkalizing effect on the rest of the body. Calcium-containing antacids are no longer popular because they tend to stimulate gastric acid secretion and may cause deposits of calcium in the soft tissues of the body.

Sometimes silicone is added to antacids as a surface tension-reducer, causing the coalescence of gas bubbles to ease their expulsion from the stomach (and thus acting as an anti-burp agent). Alginates (from seaweed) are also incorporated to produce a viscous alkaline 'raft' with the antacid, providing a mechanical barrier to prevent reflux of the stomach contents. Carminative agents, usually peppermint or similar oils, also feature in antacids to relieve flatulence and gastric colic.

Bismuth preparations:

Bismuth appears to have several modes of action on ulcer healing. These include combining with protein at the base of the ulcer, stimulating local production of ulcer-healing prostaglandins, and inhibiting the secretion and activity of the digestive enzyme pepsin. However, the most important effect is probably the rapid and profound suppression of H. pylori, which is probably what accounted for the decreased rates of relapse of duodenal ulcer in those treated with bismuth salts.

Chronic use of bismuth can cause damage to the nervous system, so treatment tends to be restricted to a maximum of eight weeks, with a similar interval before the next course of treatment. The usual dose of bismuth is 120 mg four times daily before meals, with a further 120 mg at bedtime.

Most of the bismuth components in current use are poorly soluble, which reduces their side-effects; however, excessive or prolonged use may lead to bismuth accumulation and toxicity, causing kidney failure and liver and brain damage.

An effective treatment with bismuth is when it is combined with other therapies, for example, acid-suppressive drugs and antibiotics.

Zinc:

It has been shown in animal studies that zinc can prevent the release of chemical agents which weaken the stomach lining and hence make it prone to ulceration. Zinc supplementation has been shown to accelerate the healing of peptic ulcers in people who exhibit no evidence of zinc deficiency. The usual dose is 50 mg elemental zinc taken three times daily with meals. This is a high dose for self-therapy and should be maintained only for short periods. Any potential copper deficiency induced by this amount of zinc can be prevented by taking 2 mg of copper daily. The first indication of zinc excess is diarrhoea; if this occurs, zinc supplementation should be reduced or stopped.

8

Dietary Approaches
to Peptic Ulcers

There are two types of dietary approach to peptic ulcer: one focuses on prevention, the other on curing and preventing relapse in the future.

Eat Less

Eat much less than you have been in the habit of eating. Eat simply. Make a meal of one course – one kind of mild fruit, or salad, or lightly cooked vegetables. Eat little and often. As well as being more satisfying, small, frequent meals metabolize more readily the constant production of stomach acid.

Eat sufficient protein. Experiments with laboratory animals have disclosed that if they are kept on a diet deficient in protein, 100 per cent of them develop ulcers of the duodenum or stomach. Similarly, persons with stomach or duodenal ulcers are often found to have lived on diets lacking in protein. Even when stomach ulcers in such persons have healed, they soon recur if too little protein is included in the daily diet.

Having developed a stomach ulcer, however, it cannot be healed quickly merely by increasing one's daily intake of protein. Why? Because all protein foods stimulate the flow of the gastric juices, which contain the powerful acid (hydrochloric) needed to digest proteins. This acid erodes and irritates the raw surface of the stomach ulcer, giving rise to pain. The first thing to be done, therefore, is to help nature to establish a protective coating over the ulcer and thereby expedite the healing process. To do this it is necessary to cut down one's intake of protein foods to a minimum for several weeks. This gives the ulcerous surface a respite from the irritation set up by the acid mentioned. No more than 2 or 3 oz of cheese should be taken daily during this period. It is best to omit meat altogether for the first two weeks, as meat is inferior to cheese in nutritional qualities and is not so easily digested. Wheatgerm can be used later and may be 'short-cooked' for two or three minutes in milk if desired.

Cheese:

Cheese is a more valuable form of protein than meat and has more energy value and nourishment. In addition, cheese contains lactic acid, which aids digestion and is rich in calcium – essential to strong nerves and healthy tissue. Packeted cheese is generally processed; it is advisable, therefore, to purchase unprocessed block cheese.

Take Alkaline-forming Foods

See that approximately 80 per cent of your food consists of alkaline-forming foods (fruit, raw salad vegetables, cooked vegetables, milk and dried fruits) and only 20 per cent of the acid-forming foods (meat, fish, eggs, cheese, bread, concentrated starches and sugary foods). Not alkaline powders but alkaline foods and diluted fruit juices possess the secret of neutralizing excessive acidity in the stomach, and maintaining the proper acid/alkaline balance in the blood. This is a simple, easy-to-remember principle of first-class health.

Avoid Incompatible Feeding

Avoid incompatible feeding in the following ways:

a) Don't eat a protein and a concentrated starch or sugary food at the same meal;
b) Don't eat a concentrated starch food (such as white bread and potatoes) and an acid fruit at the same meal;

c) Don't eat a milk pudding or drink milk on top of a meat meal;

d) Don't eat raw and cooked vegetables or raw and stewed fruits at the same meal.

In the case of a), b) and c), protein foods require an acid solution for their digestion. They are primarily digested by the gastric juice secreted in the stomach. All other foods require an alkaline solution for their digestion. This is secreted in the mouth and is mixed with the food in the saliva. A sick stomach cannot be both acid and alkaline at the same time. This is a difficult enough feat for a healthy stomach to achieve.

Make Good Vitamin Deficiencies

All vitamin and mineral deficiencies must be made good and maintained as a regular routine of life. Vitamins A, C, E, B_1, B_2, B_3 and the B vitamin known as pantothenic acid are great healing agents for stomach ulcers and also ulcers of the duodenum and pylorus. To save yourself having to take many tablets, a good all-round multivitamin/multimineral preparation can be taken at the rate of one tablet or capsule with each meal. A suitable formulation is one containing 100 per cent of the Recommended Daily Allowance (RDA) of all the vitamins, along with meaningful quantities of the essential minerals. (A preparation containing 100 per cent RDA of the necessary minerals would be impossible to swallow because of their sheer bulk, but as long as some minerals are present the preparation is suitable.) A high-potency prolonged release tablet taken once daily is a suitable alternative.

Extra B vitamins are needed for a variety of reasons. Persistent use of antacids, for example, particularly amongst older people, can lead to impaired absorption of vitamin B_1 with subsequent low body levels of the vitamin. It is important, therefore, to take vitamin B_1 supplements to ensure an adequate intake. Younger people are not immune either, as they too can suffer from persistent dyspepsia. One consequence of too little vitamin B_1 is constipation, so taking supplements of the vitamin whilst suffering from one gastro-intestinal complaint can prevent another.

Vitamin B_2 is needed to maintain healthy mucous membranes and it can have a preventative and curative effect on those suffering from mouth ulcers. There is no doubt that sometimes the type of person likely to suffer from peptic ulcers is also the type to develop mouth ulcers. Hence it is sound supplementation to ensure an adequate daily intake of vitamin B_2, as is true for those liable to gastric and duodenal ulcers.

When nicotinamide, or vitamin B_3 is deficient, one of the common symptoms is gastro-intestinal upsets characterized by nausea, vomiting and sometimes inflammation of the mouth and digestive tract. These symptoms, as we have seen, are also associated with gastric and duodenal ulceration, so a daily supplement of nicotinamide is a useful insurance policy.

Pantothenic acid is a B vitamin that is needed in the production of anti-stress hormones. Hence if the individual is the stressed, nervous or over-wrought type, the result can be an increased tendency to develop gastric or duodenal ulcers. Adequate pantothenic acid and, indeed, vitamin C, also will at least ensure that anti-stress hormone production is not deficient, and will lessen the tendency to produce ulcers.

Need for Fat

When insufficient fat is included in the diet, foods leave the stomach fairly rapidly and the walls of the stomach are then exposed to the action of strong hydrochloric acid for lengthy periods. We advise that a little fatty food be eaten at every meal and, after meals, a teaspoonful of olive oil be taken.

Vegetable oils are preferred to animal fats since they have protective properties not associated with the saturated animal fats. Olive oil is a rich source of the desirable monounsaturated fatty acids. Safflower or sunflower oil plus a good fish oil will supply the essential omega-6 and omega-3 polyunsaturated fatty acids respectively, both of which are needed – along with monounsaturated fatty acids – for stomach lining protection.

Vitamin A

Quite apart from the value of vitamin A in building a healthy lining to the stomach, intestines, throat and lungs, it is vitally important for resistance to all infections. In addition, though, as we have seen, high doses of this vitamin can actually heal ulcers. It is therefore quite possible that adequate intakes daily may help to prevent ulceration in the first place.

How Vitamin C Heals Ulcers

Vitamin C strengthens connective tissue and the walls of the blood vessels, both of which are essential in the healing of stomach ulcers. Dr John Marks of Downing College, Cambridge, has written in his *Guide to the Vitamins* that in gastro-intestinal disturbances vitamin C deficiency may arise through impaired absorption. The beneficial effect of vitamin C upon wound healing makes it essential that adequate amounts be administered in all cases of gastric and duodenal ulcers.

Some doctors in the US are getting remarkably good results with 1,500 mg of vitamin C daily.

However, the important thing to do is to heal the ulcer as quickly as possible. The quantity mentioned – 1,500 mg of vitamin C daily – is obtained by taking six 250-mg vitamin C tablets daily. Alternatively, this amount can be taken as a prolonged-release 1,500 mg tablet, from which the vitamin C is steadily absorbed over the whole day.

What Vitamin E Does

Animal experiments have indicated that, when subjected to stress, those animals given large amounts of vitamin E develop far fewer and less serious ulcers than those who receive nothing but a standard diet. For example, in one experiment reported in the *American Journal of Clinical Nutrition* in 1972, Dr G. F. Solomon and his colleagues compared rats that were subjected to stressful conditions. One group received 50 mg vitamin E orally twice a day along with one meal; the other group received just the one meal. After 12 days, the unsupplemented rats developed 78 per cent more ulceration than those receiving vitamin E.

It is possible that vitamin E can have a sparing effect in vitamin A deficiency. As long ago as 1946, Dr J. L. Jensen published in the journal *Science* his finding that vitamin E prevented stomach ulcers in rats receiving very low amounts of vitamin A. Later, a follow-up experiment was reported by Dr T. L. Harris and associates in the *Proceedinqs of the Society for Experimental Biology and Medicine* in 1947. Forty young rats were placed on a diet deficient in both vitamins A and E, which is known to produce ulcers. After two weeks, all rats were given vitamin A but only half of them received vitamin E. After seven weeks the rats were examined for stomach lesions. One half, those receiving just extra vitamin A, had developed stomach ulcers. Not one animal in the group receiving extra vitamin E showed any sign of ulceration.

We know that vitamin E strengthens muscular tissue and improves blood circulation. However, it also appears to help vitamin A to function, in part by protecting it, so perhaps it is not surprising that vitamin E has remarkable healing properties in ulcerous conditions.

Ensure a Good Intake of Fibre

At one time a low-fibre (or low-residue) diet was recommended in those prone to stomach problems because of the mistaken belief that the harsh, insoluble fibres would scar the stomach lining. This is no longer accepted, and the trend is now to ensure sufficient fibre in the diet, particularly the soluble kind. Soluble fibre, by thickening the stomach contents in the presence of water, slows down gastric emptying. Increasing dietary fibre has not been shown to promote the healing of peptic ulcers but it has been proved that fibres from whole grains and vegetables can help to prevent the ulcers from recurring.

High-fibre foods are the best way to increase fibre content in the diet, but it is possible to obtain soluble vegetable fibres as granules. These must be taken only after dissolving them in water to produce a gel which is easily swallowed. Never swallow dried soluble fibre preparations and never take them as tablets. In these forms, soluble fibre can swell in the throat or oesophagus, causing problems swallowing. In solution with water, such problems do not occur. High-fibre diets will ensure healthy bowel movements. This is important because the use of laxatives is to be avoided at all costs, since these drugs can also irritate the stomach lining, leading to peptic ulceration.

Avoid Certain Food Items

Caffeine – present in tea, coffee, cocoa and some soft drinks – may irritate the stomach lining and increase the chances of developing peptic ulceration. Caffeine does this by increasing acid secretion. Refined sugars in high quantities increase the risk of developing peptic ulcers by virtue of their acid-secreting property. Honey does not cause this effect, probably because the sugar has been pre-digested by the bee, and so is preferred to highly refined cane or beet sugar.

Excessive intakes of all condiments should be avoided. Highly spiced foods may irritate the stomach lining and then predispose to peptic ulceration.

Food sensitivities, including those due to allergies, appear to contribute to the chances of developing peptic ulceration. Over 50 years ago a research team showed that reactive foods slowed down stomach emptying time and caused severe swelling and redness in the stomach lining. Hence if you are aware of any food likely to cause allergy or sensitivity in your digestive system, you must avoid it.

Respiratory tract sensitivities may also be an indication of a potential peptic ulcer sufferer. In one study, 98 per cent of people with X-ray evidence of peptic ulcer also had respiratory tract allergies, suggesting that development of the ulcer may be an allergic manifestation. Microscopic study of tissues at the edge of ulcers showed evidence of a localized allergic reaction. Deliberate challenge tests of the stomach lining of those with proven food allergies indicated a direct response including swelling, erosions and bleeding in the stomach lining. This happened even in those whose skin and blood tests for allergy proved negative, suggesting that the allergenic foods were harming the stomach lining by direct action on it. Most people soon become aware of foods that upset them, and can take the necessary steps to avoid them.

Avoid Aspirin

The frequent use of aspirin, in powder or tablet form, is responsible for a good deal of stomach irritation which can later develop into stomach ulcers. However, this can be reduced by ensuring that vitamin C is taken along with aspirin. For many years it has been known that aspirin causes over-excretion of vitamin C and hence its loss from the body, and may even contribute to its destruction. Vitamin C levels are reduced by chronic ingestion of aspirin as in some arthritic and rheumatic conditions. Now it has been proved in clinical trials that supplementary vitamin C improves the absorption of aspirin, replenishes the vitamin lost by the action of the drug, reduces the irritant action of aspirin on the gastric lining, and enhances the pain-relieving properties of aspirin. Other non-steroidal anti-inflammatories used in arthritis have effects similar to those of aspirin. These effects are also reduced with supplementary vitamin C. It is important that vitamin C is taken at the same time as aspirin and the other drugs to obtain maximum benefit. The usual intake is 50–100 mg vitamin C with each aspirin or other tablet.

The Virtue of Potatoes:

Dr L. J. Nye has pointed out that stomach ulcer is almost unknown in Ireland; he relates this to the fact that potatoes appear frequently in the Irish diet. Dr

Nye recommends that stomach ulcer patients take two potato meals a day. Potatoes mashed in milk can be taken by themselves as 'mid-meals'. Potatoes contain significant amounts of vitamin C and trace elements. Ulcer patients should ensure that the potatoes they eat are baked or boiled in their skins, as otherwise much of their nutritional value is lost in cooking. Although potatoes are classified as a starchy food, they must not be confused with the factory-processed and refined starches referred to elsewhere in this book, which are of dubious food value.

Smoking and Alcohol:

There is now ample evidence of the deleterious effects of smoking on various body systems, and evidence is building up that the habit may also harm the stomach. For example, faster healing rates of gastric ulcer have been reported in those patients who gave up smoking compared to those who continued to smoke. The rate of recurrence of duodenal ulcers has been found to be significantly higher in smokers than in non-smokers. In one reported study, non-smoking had the same effect on relapse frequency as did the preventative treatment with an acid-suppressing drug. However, there is still no direct hard evidence that smokers suffer more peptic ulcers than non-smokers. The benefits seem to appear when smokers with peptic ulcers give up the habit.

A similar situation holds with drinking alcohol. Whilst excessive drinking must be discouraged to avoid alcoholic liver disease, there is no evidence that complete abstinence is a condition required for ulcer healing.

Dietary Suggestions for Treating Ulcers, Gastritis and Hiatus Hernia

The first generally-accepted and until recently widely-used dietary approach was that introduced by Dr Bertram W. Sippy, an American physician, in 1915. He used foods to neutralize excess gastric acidity, so helping the ulcer to heal naturally. Although the Sippy diet, which consisted mainly of taking milk and cream every two hours, has virtually disappeared as a treatment of peptic ulcers in developed countries, it represented the first logical dietary therapy for peptic ulcers. Its main disadvantages were that it was monotonous, likely to cause mild deficiency of some vitamins and minerals, and provided for no feeding at night. For these reasons various modifications were introduced over the years. The principle behind these dietary suggestions is to buffer gastric acidity by providing several meals per day of palatable, non-irritating foods.

Foods that are allowed include milk, cream, prepared cereals (farina, cream of wheat, strained oatmeal, puffed rice), polyunsaturated margarine, wholemeal bread, eggs, cooked fruits and vegetables, bananas (at certain times, see below), fruit juices, very lean meats (beef, lamb), fresh fish, cream or cottage cheese, custards, tapioca, rice or cornstarch pudding and plain cake made with wholewheat flours. Multivitamin supplementation is essential.

Foods to avoid include fried or highly seasoned food, spices, carbonated beverages, coffee, alcohol, meat broths, strong cheeses, coarse cereals or bread, raw fruits and vegetables (in the early stages of the complaint), rich desserts, pastry, nuts, olives and popcorn.

A typical sample diet is as follows:

Breakfast:

Wheatgerm with milk or sugar; egg, bread with polyunsaturated margarine: jelly; milk; strained fruit juices.

Lunch:

Clear soup; lean meat; potato, rice or noodles; bread with polyunsaturated margarine; jelly; milk; strained fruit juices.

Dinner:

Lean meat, fish or fowl; potato; two strained cooked vegetables; bread with polyunsaturated margarine; dessert; milk; strained fruit juices.

(Milk may be taken at any time between meals and at bedtime).

Gastro-intestinal Tract Irritability

This diet is taken to spare the gastro-intestinal tract by frequent small feedings of easily digested low-residue nutrients. The content is sugars, milk, eggs, lean meat (beef, lamb, or chicken), fish, cooked refined cereals, enriched bread, polyunsaturated margarine, cottage or cream cheese, strained cooked fruits and vegetables (or juices), potatoes, bouillon, broth, clear soups, pasta, custards, dairy ice-cream, gelatine, milk puddings, plain cake.

For a low-residue diet it is important to avoid highly seasoned or fried foods (to prevent irritation), whole or raw fruits and vegetables, wholegrain cereals and bread, bran corn, dried legumes, port, excessive fat, nuts, jams and marmalade.

Strict Diet for Ulcer Sufferers

When ulcer symptoms are severe the following diet inhibits and neutralizes gastric acid secretions and relieves pain.

Step 1:

Give 3 oz (90 ml) of cold or chilled skimmed milk or milk drinks hourly between 7 am and 9 pm.

The drink may also be continued throughout the night if there is difficulty in sleeping.

Step 2:

Continue the hourly milk feedings and gradually add egg and finely-ground cereal so that the patient is receiving egg instead of milk at 7 am and 7 pm. At 10 am, 1 pm and 4 pm, 3 oz (85 g) of cooked cereal should replace the milk.

Step 3:

A soft diet that provides essential nutrients in a form that is low in residue, well tolerated and easily digested. Suitable foods are strained soups and vegetables; fine wheat, corn or rice cereals; breads; cooked fruit (without skin or seeds); ripe bananas, grapefruit or orange sections; fresh fruit juices; potatoes; rice; ground beef; fish, fowl; eggs; cottage or cream cheese; milk; custards; gelatine; tapioca; milk puddings; ice-cream; plain cake.

Supplementary iron and other minerals, preferably as the well-absorbed amino acid chelates plus multivitamin supplements, are essential in these diets if the strict regime is continued for an extended time. Foods that must be avoided include raw fruits and vegetables, coarse breads and cereals, rich desserts, strong spices, veal, pork, all fried foods, nuts and raisins.

Diet and Vitamin Therapy for Peptic Ulcers and Acidity

Here is a suggested diet for stomach ulcer and acidity:

First Day

On rising:

Glass of milk (to be sipped slowly) with four B complex vitamin tablets.

Pre-breakfast:

Vitamin A (2,500 iu)
Vitamin B_1 (10 mg)
B complex (10 mg)
vitamin C (250 mg)
vitamin E (100 mg)
1 teaspoonful olive oil

or

A high-potency multivitamin containing 100 per cent of the Recommended Daily Allowance (RDA) of all the vitamins, along with meaningful quantities of the essential minerals.

Breakfast:

Three or more dessertspoons of a reputable brand of wheatgerm, and as much milk as you can tolerate without setting up a catarrhal condition. Soak the wheatgerm in milk (warm, if preferred) for five minutes before eating. If you prefer, the wheatgerm can be 'shortcooked' for two or three minutes in milk. For flavouring or sweetening, use honey only. If this isn't enough for some appetites, the wheatgerm and milk may be followed by fresh or dried apricots and milk or cream. Alternatively a small quantity of grapes. As the condition improves, you can follow the wheatgerm and milk with ripe peaches, or grated apple and milk, or ripe or stewed apricots.

Note: Wheatgerm is not a starch, but a protein.

Mid-morning:

Two teaspoons of brewer's yeast powder in a little milk. Alternatively, a thin slice of bread, butter and honey. If, however, you don't take the yeast at mid-morning, it should be taken at 4 o'clock or before retiring.

Before lunch:

The same vitamins as taken pre-breakfast (unless a high-potency slow-release multivitamin was taken); 1 teaspoonful of olive oil.

Lunch:

Two lightly poached eggs – no bread. Followed by grapes; if in season, or papaya. Do not eat bananas at this meal. Bananas are excellent by themselves or with other starch foods, but not with protein (eggs, meat, fish, cheese and nuts are protein).

Before the evening meal:

The same vitamins as taken pre-breakfast (unless a high-potency slow-release multivitamin was taken); 1 pantothenic acid tablet and 1 teaspoonful of olive oil.

Evening meal:

A plate of pureed vegetables – such as peas, beans, carrots, parsnips, spinach, pumpkin, cauliflower, etc. Without meat or fish, a plate of steamed vegetables is made more attractive by the addition of cheese sauce or butter sauce. Such a meal may be followed by the mild fruits, such as grapes, peaches, papaya or banana-cream puree. If you have a juice extractor, carrot, cabbage or beetroot juice is excellent for ulcers and health. Between meals, sip a glass of milk.

Second Day

Pre-breakfast:

Same as for First Day.

Breakfast:

Same as for First Day, or varied only as suggested.

Lunch:

3 oz (85 g) cheese with celery. Alternatively, cheese and ripe peaches. Later on, when the ulcer has healed, make cheese and apple, or a cheese salad, your standard lunch.

Evening meal:

Poached egg and vegetables – cooked as suggested. By way of a change, about every fourth night a little grilled fish (but no potato or bread), followed by mild, ripe fruits only (no bananas).

Vitamin and mineral supplementation as well as olive oil and the polyunsaturated oils mentioned above under 'Need for Fat' (see page 138) are essential in all these diets. Advice on these is given in the previous section (see pages 117–32).

The Healing Diet

To sum up the basic healing diet for peptic ulcers and other gastro-intestinal problems, the following considerations should apply:

Eat a wide variety of foods. The greater the spectrum of colours in your intake of fruit and vegetables, the better. There must be ample portions of fruits and vegetables (some uncooked), and wholegrain foods in the daily diet.

You should limit total fat intake to a maximum of 30 per cent of your daily calories. Daily intake of calories can be calculated using the following calorie counts: 1 gram of carbohydrate (starch), sugar or protein provides 4 calories; 1 gram of any fat or oil provides 9 calories; 1 gram of alcohol provides 7 calories. If you eat a typical Western diet, this means that you should reduce your daily fat intake by at least one quarter. Saturated fat should be limited to less than 10 per cent of the total daily calorie intake. This means a mild to moderate reduction of fat in the typical Western diet.

All vegetable oils will provide the same number of calories per gram as saturated animal fats, so ensure that the rest of your total fat intake is in the oil form. Nuts, seeds and olives are good sources of these essential dietary oils. Edible oils rich in desirable polyunsaturated and monounsaturated fatty acids include arachis (peanut), canola, corn, cottonseed, olive, safflower, sunflower, sesame and soybean.

Although there is no known direct relationship between cholesterol intake and peptic ulcers, for general health and healing you should reduce cholesterol intake to less than 300 mg daily. In a typical Western diet you will need to reduce your intake by one third.

Cholesterol-rich foods are the following: eggs – 270 mg each; fried beef liver – 600 mg per 100 g (3.5 oz); boiled shrimp – 240 mg per 100 g; pork ribs – 150 mg per 100 g; any hard cheese (e.g. cheddar) – 120 mg per 100 g.

Protein-rich foods such as red meat, fish or fowl should be no more than 120 grams (4 oz) per meal. There must be restrictions on refined sugar and salt. There is usually enough sodium already present in foods to satisfy daily needs. If you must add salt, keep it in moderation.

Alcohol intake should be restricted to 2 units per day. One unit is provided in a half-pint of beer, cider or lager; a single measure of spirits; a single glass of red or white wine; a single measure of fortified wines such as sherry, port or vermouth.

Highly salted foods and those that are smoked or charcoal-broiled should be kept to a minimum (eaten only occasionally). Most important is to control your intake of food in order to maintain a desirable body weight.

Once the ulcer has healed, the dietary advice given previously (see pages 146–150) should be adhered to. This will prevent recurrence of the ulcer and other gastric conditions.

Index

achlorhydia 76, 85
acid-suppressive drugs, and
    cancer 102–4
acidity, diet for 150–3
alcohol 145–6
alkaline powders 74–5
alkaline-forming foods 135
Aloe vera 123–4
aluminium utensils 66–7
amino acids 16
antacids 129–31
antibiotics 28–9
anticholinergics 98–9
    combined therapy with
    99–100
aspirin 144

bismuth preparations 131–2

cabbage juice 120
caffeine 142
cancers 85–6, 102–4
cheese 134–5
chewing 11
chyme 23
condiments 71–2, 143

dietary fibre, importance of
    30–1, 141–2
dietary treatment 117–18,
    146–55
digestive tract, composition
    of 11
duodenum 23–5
dyspepsia 33, 51
dysphagia 45, 50

eating habits:
  bad 70–1
  good 133–45
endoscopy 61–2

faeces 29–30
fats 15–16, 138–9
fibre *see* dietary fibre
food combinations,
  incompatible 68
  avoidance 135–6
food digestion 11–13, 17
food sensitivities 143
food transit time 12–13

garlic 121
gastritis, acute 48–9
  symptoms of 49
gastritis, chronic 50–1
gastritis, corrosive 49–50

Harris, Dr T. L. 140–1
Harrison, Dr Richard 65
Hay, Dr William Howard 74
healing diet 153–5
heartburn 38–40
Helicobacter pylori:
  action of 91–2
  discovery 89–90
  effect, and ulcers 92–3
  eradiation 94–6
  infection, prevalence 90–1
  and vitamins 96–7

herbal remedies 121–4
hiatus hernia 46–8
histamine H$_2$ receptor
  blocking agents 83, 101
hydrochloric acid:
  deficiency of 84
  increased secretion of
  80–3
  necessity of 79–80
  production of 77–8
hyperacidity 76
hypoacidity 76

indigestion:
  chronic 37–8
  nervous 36–7
  simple 32–6
irritable gastro-intestinal tract,
  diet for 148

Jensen, Dr J. L. 140
large intenstine 27–31
laxatives 73–4
lifestyle factors 9–10
liquorice 109–10
  deglycyrrhizinated 110,
  118–19
location of ulcers 61–2

Marks, Dr John 139
Marshall, Dr Barry 89–90
minerals:
  deficiencies 68–70

supplementation 129–32
Montague, Dr Joseph F. 60
mouth 18–19

nitrosamines 85–7
Nye, Dr L. J. 144

oesophagitis 42–4
    symptoms of 44–5
oesophagus 19–21
overeating 65

peptic ulcer:
    cause of 64–75
    definition of 54–7
    symptoms of 58–61
    types of 62–3
peristalsis 19
potatoes 144–5
prevention, dietary approach
    133–46
progress, results of 10
prostglandins 107–8
protein, and ulcers 67
proton pump inhibitors
    106–7
ptyalin 18

recurrence, of ulcers 104–6

salivation 17
self-therapy, with OTC drugs
    101–2

Sippy, Dr Bertram W. 146
Sippy diet 146–7
Slippery Elm Bark 122–3
small intestine 25–7
smoking 145
Solomon, Dr G. F. 140
starch, and ulcers 67
Steer, Howard 89
stomach 21–3
stress 63
    drug treatment 110–11
sucralfate 100
sugar consumption 72–3, 142
surgical operations 111–16
symphytum 122
symptoms, of peptic ulcer
    58–61

ulcer sufferers 52–4
    strict diet for 148–50

vitamin A 124–6, 139
vitamin B 136–8
vitamin C 126–7, 139–40
vitamin deficiencies 68–70,
    96–7
    making good 136–41
vitamin E 127–8, 140–1
vitamin therapy:
    and diet for peptic ulcers
    150–3
    and *Helicobacter pylori*
    96–7

warning signs 11
Warren, Dr Robin 89
'wind' 41–2

worry 65–6

zinc 132